Artificial Intelligence in Radiation Therapy

Online at: https://doi.org/10.1088/978-0-7503-3339-9

About the Series

The series in Physics and Engineering in Medicine and Biology will allow the Institute of Physics and Engineering in Medicine (IPEM) to enhance its mission to 'advance physics and engineering applied to medicine and biology for the public good'.
It is focused on key areas including, but not limited to:

- clinical engineering
- diagnostic radiology
- informatics and computing
- magnetic resonance imaging
- nuclear medicine
- physiological measurement
- radiation protection
- radiotherapy
- rehabilitation engineering
- ultrasound and non-ionising radiation.

A number of IPEM–IOP titles are being published as part of the EUTEMPE Network Series for Medical Physics Experts.

A full list of titles published in this series can be found here: https://iopscience.iop.org/bookListInfo/physics-engineering-medicine-biology-series.

Artificial Intelligence in Radiation Therapy

Edited by
Iori Sumida
Physics and Clinical Support, Accuray Japan K.K., Tokyo, Japan
and
Department of Radiation Oncology, Osaka University Graduate School of Medicine, Osaka, Japan

IOP Publishing, Bristol, UK

ISBN 978-0-7503-3339-9 (ebook)
ISBN 978-0-7503-3337-5 (print)
ISBN 978-0-7503-3340-5 (myPrint)
ISBN 978-0-7503-3338-2 (mobi)

DOI 10.1088/978-0-7503-3339-9

Version: 20221201

IOP ebooks

British Library Cataloguing-in-Publication Data: A catalogue record for this book is available from the British Library.

Published by IOP Publishing, wholly owned by The Institute of Physics, London

IOP Publishing, No.2 The Distillery, Glassfields, Avon Street, Bristol, BS2 0GR, UK

US Office: IOP Publishing, Inc., 190 North Independence Mall West, Suite 601, Philadelphia, PA 19106, USA

Contents

Preface

John McCarthy is an American computer scientist and inventor, who developed 'artificial intelligence' in 1956 to explore ways to make computers behave like humans, e.g., thinking, problem-solving, and self-improvement. Since then, computer power has been growing with the improvement in performance of central processing units (CPU) and graphical processing units (GPU). Based on the technical improvements, artificial intelligence (AI) could develop to a level which is close to that of human thought processes. To develop AI to that level much trial and error will be necessary to fine tune the machine learning process and modify the neural network. Big data for training AI will also be necessary.

This textbook provides applications of AI in radiation therapy according to the clinical radiotherapy workflow. An introductory section explains the necessity for AI with regard to accuracy and efficiency in clinical work. This is followed by a basic learning method, and the introduction of potential applications in radiotherapy. For many people in the radiotherapy field that have not followed the development of AI applications, this textbook will provide a comprehensive overview of the topics and will demonstrate the practical skills/knowledge of implementing/using the developed application. It will also be useful to more experienced practitioners and researchers and members of medical physics communities. Since some chapters include or link to some typical source codes which will contribute to clinical areas, the book could be useful for students who are focusing on medical physics.

I am grateful to the chapter authors, who are world renowned experts and scientists in the field of radiation therapy. I acknowledge Michael Slaughter (Senior Commissioning Editor), Emily Tapp (Commissioning Editor), and Sarah Armstrong (Editorial Assistant), for their valuable help in making this publication possible. Finally, I am very greatful to Indra J Das who is my advisor for handling the book.

Iori Sumida
Physics and Clinical Support, Accuray Japan K.K., Tokyo, Japan
Department of Radiation Oncology, Osaka University, Osaka, Japan

Editor biography

Iori Sumida

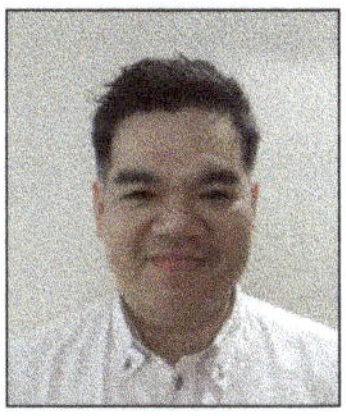

Iori Sumida is a Director of Physics and clinical support in Accuray Japan K.K. and is also an invited faculty of Department of Radiation Oncology, Osaka University Graduate School of Medicine, Japan as a cross appointment. Dr Sumida earned his BSc and MSc degrees in Health Sciences in 1999 and 2001, respectively. He earned his PhD in Radiation Oncology from Osaka University in 2005. His qualifications are radiation technologist as a national license in Japan and a medical physicist accredited by Japanese Board of Medical Physicist (JBMP) Qualification. He is a committee member of the JBMP, Japan Society of Medical Physics (JSMP), Japanese Society for Radiation Oncology (JASTRO), The Japanese College of Medical Physics (JCMP), and Computer Assisted Radiology and Surgery (CARS) in charge of representative and councilor. Dr Sumida has almost two decades of hands-on experience in the field of quality assurance and treatment planning in medical physics and has software development skill to dedicate and to contribute making radiotherapy accurate and precise. He has authored or coauthored more than 100 technical articles (102 journals, 8 books, and one book chapter).

List of contributors

Bin Cai
Department of Radiation Oncology, University of Texas Southwestern Medical Center, Dallas, TX, USA

Ibrahim Chamseddine
General Hospital, Harvard Medical School and Massachusetts General Hospital, Boston, MA, USA

Quan Chen
Department of Radiation Medicine, University of Kentucky College of Medicine, Lexington, KY, USA

Leigh Conroy
Radiation Medicine Program, Princess Margaret Cancer Centre, University of Toronto, Toronto, ON, Canada

Clemens Grassberger
General Hospital, Harvard Medical School and Massachusetts General Hospital, Boston, MA, USA

Charles Huang
Department of Radiation Oncology, Stanford University, CA, USA

Noriyuki Kadoya
Department of Radiation Oncology, Tohoku University Graduate School of Medicine, Sendai, Japan

Yejin Kim
Harvard Medical School and Massachusetts General Hospital, USA
and
Korean Advanced Institute of Science and Technology, Korea

Men Kuo
Department of Radiation Oncology, Cancer Hospital, Chinese Academy of Medical Science, Beijing, China

Tianye Niu
Nuclear and Radiological Engineering and Medical Physics Programs, Woodruff School of Mechanical Engineering, Georgia Institute of Technology, Atlanta, GA, USA

Omid Nohadani
Department of Industrial Engineering and Management Sciences, Northwestern University, Evanston, IL, USA
and
Benefits Science Technology, Boston, MA, USA

Jay Patel
Temple University College of Public Health, Philadelphia, PA, USA

X Sharon Qi
Department of Radiation Oncology, UCLA School of Medicine, Los Angeles, CA, USA

Yi Rong
Department of Radiation Oncology, Mayo Clinic, Phoenix, AZ, USA

Yang Sheng
Department of Radiation Oncology, Duke University Medical Center, Durham, NC, USA

Iori Sumida
Physics and Clinical Support, Accuray Japan K.K., Tokyo, Japan
and
Department of Radiation Oncology, Osaka University, Osaka, Japan

Yi Wang
Department of Radiation Oncology, Massachusetts General Hospital, Harvard Medical School, Boston, MA, USA

Zhichao Wang
Nuclear and Radiological Engineering and Medical Physics Programs, Woodruff School of Mechanical Engineering, Georgia Institute of Technology, Atlanta, GA, USA

Zhao Wei
School of Physics, Beihang University, Beijing, China

and
Department of Radiation Oncology, Stanford University, Palo Alto, CA, USA

Huanmei Wu
Temple University College of Public Health, Philadelphia, PA, USA

Lei Xing
Department of Radiation Oncology, Stanford University, CA, USA

Xiao Ying
Department of Radiation Oncology, University of Pennsylvania, Philadelphia, PA, USA

Jiahan Zhang
Department of Radiation Oncology, Emory University, Atlanta, GA, USA

Chapter 1

Introduction

Iori Sumida

The clinical workflow in radiotherapy is shown in figure 1.1. It can be seen that radiotherapy consists of a number of steps from simulation at the beginning to clinical evaluation at the end.

Radiation therapists, medical dosimetrists, medical physicists, and radiation oncologists are involved in each step. In the simulation process, a radiation technologist sets up the patient using an immobilization device, this is followed by the image acquisition using computed tomography and magnetic resonance imaging for the imaging process. In the treatment planning, after a radiation oncologist has delineated the target contours and prescribed the dose to the target, a medical dosimetrist and a medical physicist delineate the normal tissues and create a treatment plan. The treatment plan data is forwarded to the treatment database and is verified by a medical physicist. Finally, a radiation therapist sets up the patient and verifies the treatment position of the patient, irradiation then starts. After the radiation treatment session, a radiation oncologist conducts a clinical evaluation of the patient.

Using an advanced treatment machine with high specification, a more sophisticated imaging device for image acquisition and guidance, and a high-performance dose calculation engine for the treatment planning system, accurate radiation treatment can be delivered to the patient such as intensity-modulated radiation therapy and stereotactic radiation therapy.

To date, artificial intelligence (AI) has provided support in conducting radiotherapy workflows accurately and efficiently. The organ delineation step is a first aim for AI contribution, because it is a laborious and subjective process [1] for the treatment planners. When AI delineates the contour instead of a human, the clinical workflow can be changed efficiently. However, it is important to confirm how well AI works; this means that, because the accuracy of organ delineation directly correlates to dose calculation accuracy, i.e., dose optimization and dose evaluation, we must verify the results of the work done by AI. Second, AI supports the

doi:10.1088/978-0-7503-3339-9ch1

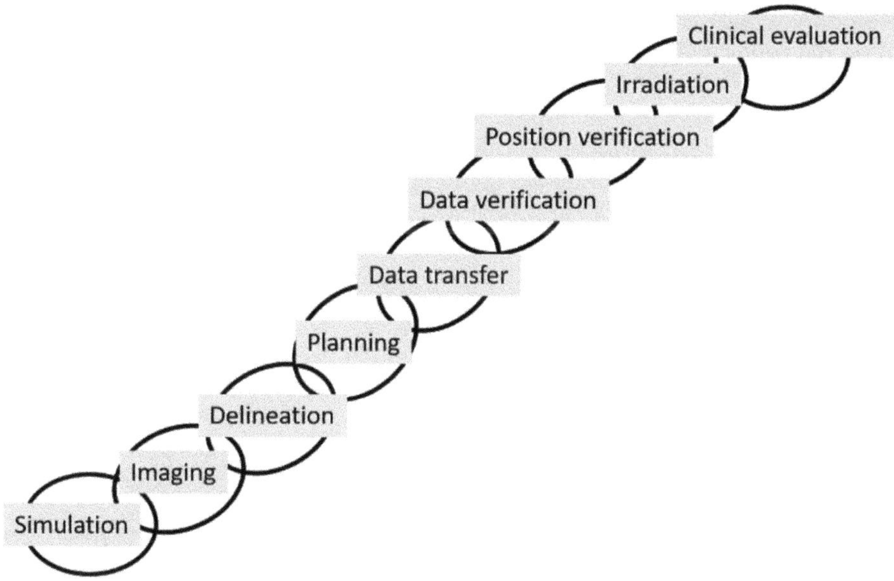

Figure 1.1. Clinical workflow in radiotherapy.

simulation step. Although research into the simulation step might be in progress, CT to MRI [2] and MRI to CT image translation [3], low-dose CT to normal dose CT translation, etc, have been adopted in this step. These focus on accurate organ delineation and reduction of radiation exposure to the patient. For example, MRI to CT image translation will help us to further oriented radiation therapy which uses only MRI for dose calculation [4]. Third, AI supports the image registration step for image guidance. Although image processing also supports image registration mathematically using an intensity-based [5] and mutual information-based [6] registration method, the calculation may take longer to perform then when performed by AI. Fourth, AI predicts the clinical outcome after radiotherapy which varies from three-dimensional radiation therapy to intensity-modulated radiation therapy and stereotactic radiotherapy, etc. The clinical outcome of the patient also depends on the patients' background such as their chemotherapy history. Therefore, diversified data is necessary to predict the clinical outcome precisely.

As mentioned above, the practitioner should use various kinds of mixed data (numerical/categorical and image data) to develop their own network which is in accordance to the purpose of the radiotherapy.

References

[1] Liu Z, Liu X and Guan H *et al* 2020 Development and validation of a deep learning algorithm for auto-delineation of clinical target volume and organs at risk in cervical cancer radiotherapy *Radiother. Oncol.* **153** 172–9

[2] Li W, Li Y and Qin W *et al* 2020 Magnetic resonance image synthesis from brain computed tomography deep learning methods for magnetic resonance (MR)-guided radiotherapy *Quant. Imaging Med. Surg.* **10** 1223–36

[3] Kearney V, Ziemer B P and Perry A *et al* 2020 Attention-aware discrimination for MR-to-CT image translation using cycle-consistent generative adversarial networks *Radiol. Artif. Intell.* **2** e190027
[4] Palmer E, Karlsson A and Nordstrom F *et al* 2021 Synthetic computed tomography data allows for accurate absorbed dose calculations in a magnetic resonance imaging only workflow for head and neck radiotherapy *Phys. Imaging Radiat. Oncol.* **17** 36–42
[5] Lee M E, Kim S H and Seo I H Intensity-based registration of medical images *2009 Int. Conf. on Test and Measurement (Hong Kong, China, 2009)* pp 239–42
[6] Pluim J P W, Maintz J B A and Viergever M A 2003 Mutual-information-based registration of medical images: a survey *IEEE Trans. Med. Imaging* **22** 986–1004

Chapter 2

Artificial intelligence and machine learning

Omid Nohadani

The success of artificial intelligence and machine learning has witnessed a steady growth over the past several decades. The recent abundance of computing power and data, both in terms of size and complexity, has accelerated this advancement to a level that these technologies are now affecting human life. This chapter gives a broad introduction to the field, starting with basic principles of learning, and establishes a framework that unifies many common methodologies. We discuss details of techniques that directly apply to recent developments in radiation therapy, such as mixture models, regression and classification models, decision trees, and neural networks.

2.1 Introduction

Learning is a basic evolutionary process of acquiring knowledge and understanding of the environment, not only in its physical meaning but also in the abstract. It can be instantaneous by a single observation or through numerous iterations of unique, yet similar, steps. Given its key role in evolution, learning can be a continuous process of improving learning strategies. When observations are quantifiable, their corresponding data can be leveraged to facilitate the learning process via computer algorithms. Such an algorithmic approach becomes essential in two settings.

The first setting is when a lack of human experience or the inability to transfer the knowledge hinders learning. An example of such a setting is the recognition of spoken language, where acoustically measurable signals need to be converted into written text. In the presence of a human listener who is fluent in that language, this task is seemingly natural. However, the absence of such expertise or complete explanation renders this task challenging. Even different people have a different understanding of the same words and further, dialects can perturb proper comprehension. In an algorithmic approach, a large collection of past spoken words from different people is mapped to written language by systematically minimizing errors.

doi:10.1088/978-0-7503-3339-9ch2

The second setting is when the underlying knowledge to be learned varies, e.g., in time or with respect to its reference environment. For instance, when the information changes faster than the human mind can arrive at a good decision. The goal is to develop an approach that can adapt to its environment and deliver reliable and sustainable insights that are independent of the respective circumstances. An example is network traffic management, when (digital) packets are routed over a network with arcs with differing levels of congestion. A learning algorithm would continuously adapt to current parameters by observing the behavior of the network or its subsets to find the optimal routing pattern.

This chapter begins with a discussion of the foundations of algorithmic learning. Given the myriad of current methods, we will first discuss them at a higher level to distinguish between *supervised*, *unsupervised*, *semi-supervised*, and *reinforcement learning* approaches. We choose the network representation to introduce common methods since it provides a unifying framework for both statistical learning as well as neural network techniques. This chapter concludes with specifics on more relevant approaches that pertain to radiation therapy.

2.1.1 Foundations, similarities, and differences

Machine Learning (ML) is programming computers for the purpose of extracting knowledge and improving performance criteria by using available data from observations or past experiences. ML is often viewed as an extension of statistical learning. However, the fundamental difference is the reliance on data models and the assumption that observed data follow probability distribution models. This difference is best highlighted by Leo Breiman who stated that 'the statistical community has been committed to the almost exclusive use of data models. This commitment has led to irrelevant theory, questionable conclusions, and has kept statisticians from working on large range and interesting current problems'. In contrast to statistical learning, ML has the capability to directly leverage results and insights of probability theory to infer knowledge, free of distributional assumptions. An illustrative example of this is the Central Limit Theorem, one of the hallmark results of probability theory, which states that the sum of normalized independent random variables converges to a normal (Gaussian) distribution, irrespective of the original distribution of the random variables. This view allows us to regard data as the only measurable manifestation of reality and to regard models as vehicles in our imagination to simplify or prescind the reality. This data-driven approach has been attributed to the wide applicability and growth of ML methods in recent decades. While many of the methods have heavily relied on heuristics, formal optimization methods have recently accelerated this progress, as will be explored in subsequent discussions.

Artificial Intelligence (AI) is the decision-making capability of machines that collect information about the environment with the goal of successfully and efficiently completing tasks. The foundation of AI is based on the assumption that human intelligence can be 'simulated'. In essence, the field of AI seeks to build machines, that think and act similarly to humans by simulating *rational* thinking and acting. In this context, the concept of rationality needs to be regarded as steps that maximally achieve pre-determined goals. Therefore, it relates only to decisions taken and not the thought process that led to that decision. As a result, the solution of an AI model may lose its humanly interpretable power. This computational rationality solely seeks to maximize the expected utility of outcomes. Although the human mind is excellent at rational decision making, its structure is not modular and, it cannot be reverse engineered into software. Nonetheless, its memory and the simulation thereof can serve as a basis for algorithmic decision making.

2.1.2 Connection to decision making

In addition to the commercial solutions that already exist for automatic speech and image recognition, ML has driven decision making in other areas such as: retail sales data informing future inventory positions and enhancing customer experience; historical financial transactions adapting lending policies; and healthcare insurance data motivating underwriting and guiding risk assessment.

In ML, decision making requires an entity called, an *agent*, which has the capability of *perception* and the potential to take *action* based on those perceptions. A *rational agent* autonomously selects actions that maximize its expected utility. In strenuous environments, agents need to learn to adjust their behavior to complete tasks with fewer resources, e.g., on a distant planet of for post-disaster relief. The parameters that describe the precepts, environment, and action space determine the methodological approach for selecting rational actions.

2.2 Overview of learning methods

In principle, learning algorithms can be grouped in different ways, e.g., by computational similarities, by underlying assumptions, or by the type of inference they provide. In this introduction, we divide them based on their learning types into *supervised, unsupervised, semi-supervised*, and *reinforcement learning* algorithms. In most approaches, the data is typically divided into a training and test set. Whether or not the data is labeled, determines which learning type is used. While supervised learning assumes the training data to be labeled, unsupervised learning takes in data that is not labeled and its outcomes are yet unknown. Semi-supervised learning, as its name suggests, acts on input data that is a mixture of labeled and unlabeled samples in both training and testing samples. In reinforcement learning, in addition to the above distinction, the outcome of the previous learning iteration is evaluated by a reward function, whose feedback is leveraged as input of the next learning iteration.

2.2.1 Supervised learning

In supervised learning, the goal is to map the input to an output whose correct values (called label or target) are provided by a supervisor who we assume has perfect knowledge. The simplest case is learning class from its positive and negative examples. This can be generalized to multiple but distinct outcomes, known as *multi-class classification*, or continuous outcomes, known as *regression* methods.

A classification algorithm will be given a set of training data vectors $\boldsymbol{x}$ with assigned labels or categories $\boldsymbol{y}$. The model finds the features within the components of $\boldsymbol{x}$ that best correlate to each class and generates a mapping function $f(\boldsymbol{x}) = \boldsymbol{x}$ for any data point $\boldsymbol{x}$. The goal is to then take unlabeled (test) data and assign it a class based on trained model f. The way the mapping function f is trained, heavily depends upon the underlying data, application, and the objective of learning. Popular algorithms in this context are linear and logistic regressions, support vector machines, decision trees, instant-based (e.g., K-nearest neighbors), and random forest algorithms. A large portion of section 2.3 is devoted to a more detailed discussion of some of these algorithms. In practice, supervised learning methods are the most commonly used approaches to ML and have proven practical to extract insights in many real-world applications.

2.2.2 Unsupervised learning

In unsupervised learning, there is no supervisor with perfect knowledge to label the data. Therefore, we are left with unlabeled input data and the goal is to find regularities in them. The assumption is that there exists a structure in the input data space which reveals itself in certain patterns more often than others and the goal is—statistically speaking—to estimate the density of these patterns. A prominent example of such density estimation is *clustering*, where clusters or groups of input data are identified. Consequently, those input data that are different than the identified clusters can be considered *outliers*. Clustering is often applied to *image compression*, where the image pixel representation in RGB values is grouped into pixels of similar colors, based on the frequency of their occurrence in the picture. The structure of the data can then be exploited to identify redundancies and determine a shortened description of the data, resulting in a compressed representation.

2.2.3 Semi-supervised learning

In semi-supervised learning, the input data contains a mixture of labeled and unlabeled examples. In this setting, while there exists a desired learning problem, the model has to learn the structures in order to both organize the data and make predictions. Prominent examples are regression and classification problems on partially labeled data. Typically, only a small fraction of data has labels, and this fraction is leveraged to improve the learning accuracy. Given that the acquisition of labels often requires human experts or actual and controlled experiments to collect labels, the availability of large sets of reliable labels is rather scarce, making semi-supervised techniques of practical importance. One of the popular set of methods in this context are *generative models*, where in the training step, the distribution of data belonging to a class is estimated, in order to then compute the probability of a given point in the test data to have a certain label. In principle, semi-supervised learning with generative models can be regarded as an extension of both the supervised and unsupervised methods.

2.2.4 Reinforcement learning

In some learning settings, there is not just one outcome but a sequence of them, also known as *actions*. What it takes to accomplish a goal is a *policy* that determines the sequence of these actions. Therefore, the objective is to access the goodness of policies and learn from past sequences of actions to inform the generation of future policies. These learning methods are typically referred to as *reinforcement learning* algorithms. In the example of a mechanical robot that has the goal of starting from an initial location and arriving at a destination, it can move in a few directions at any point in time. We expect it to learn the correct sequence of moves after some initial trials to reach the targeted destination in an efficient and safe fashion, i.e., without hitting obstacles. However, when the system receives only partial or unreliable sensory information, this task becomes increasingly harder. A task may also require multiple agents to act in a cooperative manner to reach a common goal by establishing strategic communication in constrained environments, e.g., a swarm of unmanned aerial vehicles.

2.3 Common algorithms

From the perspective of the underlying statistical model for learning from data, three broad modeling problems can be considered, namely (i) classification, (ii) regression, and (iii) density estimation, where (i) and (ii) correspond to supervised learning and (iii) refers to unsupervised learning. In general, the first two namely classification and regression problems can be viewed as special cases of density estimation, because the objective of density estimation is to estimate the unconditional distribution of the data $\boldsymbol{x}$. Interpreting x-ray images (e.g., mammograms for breast cancer screening) is a practical example of density estimation [1]. The training data $\boldsymbol{x}$ is taken from non-cancerous images and a density estimation method—in this case a network model—is employed to construct a representation of the probability density $p(\boldsymbol{x})$. When the model is applied to a new (test) image $\boldsymbol{x}'$, an increased value of $p(\boldsymbol{x}')$ suggests a non-cancerous image. On the other hand, a decreased $p(\boldsymbol{x}')$ indicates a novel observation and a potential sign of an abnormality is flagged for further clinical inspection.

To generalize this concept, the underlying data can be described by the probability distribution function $p(\boldsymbol{x}, \boldsymbol{y})$ in the joint input-target space. Given that the typical goal is to predict the target variables (classes), when exposed to new and unknown input data

$$p(\boldsymbol{x}, \boldsymbol{y}) = p(\boldsymbol{y}|\boldsymbol{x})p(\boldsymbol{x}) \tag{2.1}$$

by using only the *conditional probability* $p(\boldsymbol{y}|\boldsymbol{x})$, i.e., the distribution of $\boldsymbol{y}$ given the value of $\boldsymbol{x}$. In other words, we need the conditional densities for classification and regression. Hence, while density estimation on its own can be the objective of the learning, it is often used as a component of the solution to more general problems in classification or regression. In what follows, we use the network representation to introduce some of the common methods, as this representation naturally lends itself to unify the description of both statistical learning and neural network methods.

2.3.1 Gaussian mixture models

To introduce the concept in network representation, note that in equation (2.1) the joint distribution is composed of $p(\boldsymbol{y}|\boldsymbol{x})$ and the unconditional probability $p(\boldsymbol{x})$ for the input. The two reasons, why constructing an explicit model for $p(\boldsymbol{x})$ is useful is that it allows to (i) impute missing data in the input set, which is fairly common in real-world datasets, and (ii) estimate the joint probability $p(\boldsymbol{x},\boldsymbol{y})$ and in reverse compute the conditional density of $p(\boldsymbol{x}|\boldsymbol{y})$. This inverse probability is often used in optimization and control applications.

Consider the observed data to be a sample from a *mixture density* of M densities. This mixture density can be expressed as

$$p(\boldsymbol{x}|\boldsymbol{w}) = \sum_{i=1}^{M} \pi_i p(\boldsymbol{x}|i, \boldsymbol{w}_i). \tag{2.2}$$

The *mixing proportion* π_i is a constant and *component densities* $p(\boldsymbol{x}|i,\boldsymbol{w}_i)$ can be extracted from a simple parametric family. In the case of the multivariate Gaussian, the parameters $\boldsymbol{w}_i$ represent the mean and covariance matrices belonging to each component. By appropriately adjusting $\boldsymbol{w}_i$, these models can describe a broad range of high-dimensional and multi-model real-world problems. Notice that this approach can also be viewed as a probabilisitic clustering [2].

Figure 2.1 illustrates the network model of such a Gaussian mixture model, where the links highlight the weights μ_{ij} for the component j of the mean vector of the Gaussian i. The intermediate node i computes $p(\boldsymbol{x}|i,\mu_i,\boldsymbol{\Sigma}_i)$ using the covariance matrix $\boldsymbol{\Sigma}_i$. A wide variety of statistical models can be represented by such network representation, e.g., principle component analysis, kernel density estimation, canonical correlation analysis, and factor analysis [3].

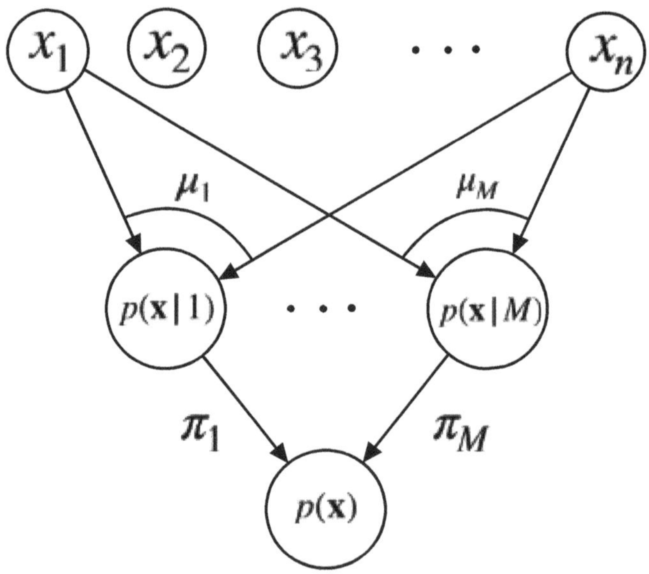

Figure 2.1. An illustration of a Gaussian mixture distribution represented by a network. Top row nodes show the input $\boldsymbol{x}$ represented by its numerical value. The output node calculates the weighted sum of the component densities $p(\boldsymbol{x}) = \sum_i \pi_i p(\boldsymbol{x}|i, \mu_i, \Sigma_i)$.

2.3.2 Regression and classification algorithms

The focus of both regression and classification methods is on computing the conditional probability $p(\boldsymbol{y}|\boldsymbol{x})$. However, these two methods differ, because in regression the outcome vector $\boldsymbol{y}$ is real-valued, while in classification $\boldsymbol{y}$ can take values from a discrete set of class labels. In this setting, a probabilistic model for regression can be constructed by $\boldsymbol{y}$ being the sum of a deterministic function $f(\boldsymbol{x})$ and some Gaussian random variable, also known as noise:

$$y = f(x) + \varepsilon \tag{2.3}$$

Notice that $f(\boldsymbol{x})$ becomes the *conditional expected value* $E(\boldsymbol{y}|\boldsymbol{x})$, whenever ε can be assumed to have a zero mean, which is often the case. More general regression models can also provide higher moments than the first moment, described by $E(\boldsymbol{y}|\boldsymbol{x})$.

The simplest regression model, namely *linear regression* assumes the conditional expectation to be a linear function of $\boldsymbol{x}$ via $E(\boldsymbol{y}|\boldsymbol{x}) = \boldsymbol{W}\boldsymbol{x}$ for a pre-determined matrix $\boldsymbol{W}$. Translated to the network representation of figure 2.1, in a linear regression the input j represents component j of the input vector x_j, each output i is computed by the weighted sum of x_j, weighted by w_{ij} placed on the link between input j and output i.

In classification problems, in addition to the conditional expectation, a *discriminant function* plays a key role. To showcase its importance, consider a two-class problem with binary outcomes $y \in \{0,1\}$. Consequently, the conditional expectation becomes the probability of $y = 1$, which can be computed using Bayes' rule

$$p(y = 1|\mathrm{x}) = \frac{p(\mathrm{x}|y = 1)p(y = 1)}{p(\mathrm{x}|y = 1)p(y = 1) + p(\mathrm{x}|y = 0)p(y = 0)} \tag{2.4}$$

where $p(y|\boldsymbol{x})$ is often referred to as the *posterior probability* of the class given the input, $p(\boldsymbol{x}|y)$ as the *class-conditional density*, and the denominator is the expansion of $p(\boldsymbol{x})$. To show the connection to regression models, we can rewrite equation (2.4) as

$$p(y = 1|\mathrm{x}) = \frac{1}{1 + \exp\left(-\ln\left[\frac{p(\mathrm{x}|y = 1)}{p(\mathrm{x}|y = 0)}\right] - \ln\left[\frac{p(y = 1)}{p(y = 0)}\right]\right)} \tag{2.5}$$

which allows us to express the *posterior* probability via the *logistic function* $g(z)$, where z is a function of the likelihood ratio $p(\boldsymbol{x}|y = 1)/p(\boldsymbol{x}|y = 0)$ and the prior ratio $p(y = 1)/p(y = 0)$:

$$g = \frac{1}{1 + e^{-z}} \tag{2.6}$$

When z takes a simple form, which is often the case in classification problems, then this becomes a useful representation of the *posterior* probability. Interestingly, z becomes a linear function of $\boldsymbol{x}$ as $z = w^{\mathrm{T}}\boldsymbol{x} + \omega_0$, when the class-conditional densities are multivariate Gaussians with identical covariance matrices, i.e., independent and identically normal distributed, which is a common assumption. Moreover, this representation can also be applied to the broad family of exponential probability distributions, such as the Gaussian, the Poisson, the gamma, the binomial, etc, because distributions in this class all exhibit the form

$$\rho(\mathrm{x}; \boldsymbol{\theta}, \phi) = \exp\left(\frac{\boldsymbol{\theta}^{\mathrm{T}}\mathbf{x} - b(\boldsymbol{\theta})}{a(\phi)} + c(\mathbf{x}, \phi)\right) \tag{2.7}$$

where $\boldsymbol{\theta}$ and ϕ denote the location and scale parameter, respectively. Using this formulation, we can derive that z is a linear function in all cases, when we insert (2.7) into equation (2.5) and allow $\boldsymbol{\theta}$ to vary between the classes while keeping ϕ constant between the classes.

Discriminant functions, such as in the example of z above, can be employed to make a decision on class membership [4]. In the example so far, we have generated a discriminant function that serves as an intermediate step to compute the *posterior* probability. When $z = 0$, the boundary of the logistic function yields $p = 0.5$. That means, $z = 0$ establishes the *decision boundary* separating the two binary classes.

When the class-conditional density functions are more complex than the above linear setting with the conditions on ϕ and a single exponential family density, the *posterior* probability cannot be uniquely characterized by the linear-logistic form. Nevertheless, the field of neural networks takes the useful step of still retaining the logistic function and focusing on *nonlinear representations* for z.

While linear models can be viewed as restrictive by the strong linearity assumption, their simplicity gives rise to practical benefits. From a geometrical viewpoint, the linear function $\boldsymbol{w}^{\mathrm{T}}\boldsymbol{x} + \omega_0$ in $\boldsymbol{x}$ space with $\boldsymbol{x}$ is constant on all hyperplanes that are orthogonal to $\boldsymbol{w}$, allowing predictable power.

2.3.2.1 Nonlinear regression and classification algorithms

In many applications, a more general function is required for a more accurate representation. Here, we discuss nonlinear mappings that enable approximations of any given mapping at a high accuracy. There are several approaches that can serve this purpose, and we consider a transformation of the input data $\boldsymbol{x}$ via a set of M nonlinear functions $\phi_j(\boldsymbol{x})$ with 1, 2, …, M. Parallel to the network representation in the previous section, we can form a linear combination of these functions

$$g_k(\boldsymbol{x}) = \sum_j w_{kj}\phi_j(\boldsymbol{x}). \tag{2.8}$$

This model can achieve a sufficient approximation for a large enough M and a suitable choice of the functions $\phi_j(\boldsymbol{x})$. In the case of an input space with $d = 1$, $\phi_j(\boldsymbol{x})$ can be constructed by a simple polynomial of successive powers of x, where the parameter w becomes the polynomial coefficient. This model can be represented in a network fashion by a single layer of adaptive weights.

In general, it is important to have significantly more data points than adaptive parameters in order to achieve a reliable generalization. A challenge in this context is the so-called *curse of dimensionality*, e.g., for a polynomial of order M, the number of independent coefficients that need to be determined grows as d^M [5]. However, in many real-world problems, one can find strong correlations between the input features (dimensions) that prevent the data to completely fill the input space. Therefore, it often becomes sufficient to confine the model to a sub-space of the data, also known as *intrinsic dimensionality*. In equation (2.8), the basis functions $\phi_j(\boldsymbol{x})$ can become *adaptive* via internal weight parameters which can be adjusted once the data is observed.

When the basis function is given by linear-logistic functions as in equation (2.6), they are called *multilayer perceptron* (MLP) [2]. The corresponding multivariate nonlinear function can then be given by

$$g_k(\mathrm{x}) = \sum_{j=1}^{M} \omega_{kj} h\left(\sum_{i=1}^{d} \omega_{ji} x_i + \omega_{j0} \right) + \omega_{k0} \tag{2.9}$$

where w_{j0} and w_{k0} are *bias* parameters. In this context, the basis functions are known as *hidden units*. These functions build the foundation of neural networks, as we will discuss later. Connecting to equation (2.6), function $h(\cdot)$ is the corresponding logistic sigmoid function, and the network representation can be sketched as in figure 2.2. In such a network representation, the data dimensionality is directly built in via the first layer of weights w_{ji}, which can align the surface such that the basic function value becomes constant. When the number of hidden units M is sufficiently large, these models can approximate any continuous function with high accuracy. This is called a compact domain. These MLP models can be extended to also accommodate multiple layers of weights.

When, on the other hand, the basis function $\phi_j(\boldsymbol{x})$ in equation (2.8) can be expressed via a distance to some a moment, say $\boldsymbol{x} - \mu_j$ with μ_j the center of the $\phi_j(\boldsymbol{x})$, then the corresponding network model is expressed by a *radial basis function* (RBF). A Gaussian distribution with the adaptive mean μ_j and covariance matrix $\boldsymbol{\Sigma}_j$ can be used to express a popular form of the basis function via

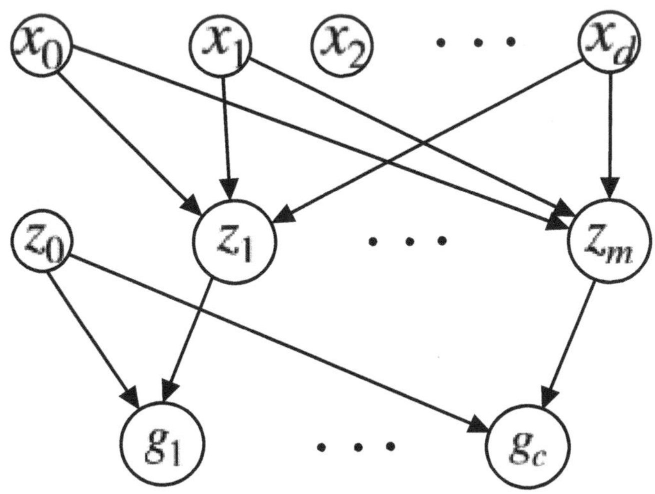

Figure 2.2. Illustration of a feed-forward network: top row shows the input units x_i and the bottom row shows the output units g_k. The bias parameters for activation are set to be for the input layer $x_0 = 1$ and for the second layer $z_0 = 1$, where $z_{i\geqslant 1}$ are the weights of the hidden units.

$$\phi_j(\mathbf{x}) = \exp\left(-\frac{1}{2}(\mathbf{x} - \boldsymbol{\mu}_j)^{\mathrm{T}} \sum_j^{-1} \mathbf{x} - \boldsymbol{\mu}_j\right) \tag{2.10}$$

Notice that $\phi_j(\boldsymbol{x})$ can be positioned and rotated in the $\boldsymbol{x}$ space in order to overlay the sections of high data density with the goal to describe potential correlations amongst the input features. This means that the number of free parameters in this model does not grow with dimensionality, i.e., the curse of dimensionality is lifted. An efficient way to train such an RBF network consists of two stages, where first the basic function parameters are computed by estimating the density of a mixture model on the training data. Here, $\phi_j(\boldsymbol{x})$ can be used as the components of the density function. The basis function parameters then remain constant in the second stage, and the second-layer weights w_{kj} are determined by minimizing the standard least squares [5].

While MLP and RBF networks share a common construction from adaptive basis functions, they differ in the support of their basis function. More specifically, the linear-logistic basis functions of MLP networks are bounded away from zero for an extended section of the input space $\boldsymbol{x}$. That means, that each input vector potentially contributes towards a distributed pattern over the hidden units of an MLP network model, supporting the notion of a 'global network.' In contrast, RBF networks are regarded as 'local', because their Gaussian basis functions are typically supported only over a subregion of the $\boldsymbol{x}$ space. Note that this support, despite its local nature, does not imply non-overlapping. To this end, another family of models with basis functions that have non-overlapping support is *decision trees*, which we will discuss next.

2.3.3 Decision-tree algorithms

A decision tree is in principle a regression or classification model and can be constructed via a sequence of linear questions (or decisions) that dissects the $\boldsymbol{x}$ space [6]. The series of questions allow us to systematically dissect input data into smaller partitions in a recursive fashion. Simply put, each question can take the form of 'is $x_i < c$ or $x_i \geqslant c$?' for some value of c. As a result, all input vectors that end up in a *leaf* of the tree span a polyhedral region, whose collection constitutes a set of basis functions. Consequently, each of these functions provides an output value. For regression methods, this value corresponds to the average of the conditional mean, or for classification it relates to a discriminant function or the majority votes within the leaf. Therefore, the output can be expressed as a weighted sum of the basis functions.

In general, decision trees and MLP/RBF neural networks reside on the same continuum of modeling approaches. All these models have overlapping or non-overlapping basis functions. In fact, it was shown that decision trees can be expressed in a probabilistic manner as mixture models and that in the mixture approaches the smoothing of the rather sharp boundaries of discriminant function for trees results in a partially-overlapping basis function [2].

A very important aspect of decision trees is that their results are *interpretable*, which is a key advantage of decision trees of other ML approaches. In many applications, in particular in healthcare, the interpretability of the outcomes is preferred over small improvements in the accuracy of other methods that have less-interpretable results. Clinical practitioners arrive at their judgment by considering one variable at a time, making decision trees more consistent with human thinking.

2.3.3.1 Classification and regression trees

The method of *classification and regression trees* (CART) is a prominent example of interpretable methods [7, 8]. It partitions from the root node and a split is recursively computed by optimizing for the best split prior to actually splitting the data based on this split. CART determines the best split by measuring the label similarity of data points within each group and by minimizing the sum of dis-similarities within each group. For classification problems, the typical measure is the *Gini* or *towing criteria* and for regression the *mean squared error* or *mean absolute error* [9].

The efficacy of CART due to its interpretability is somewhat tampered with by its less competitive level of accuracy, when compared to tailored ML methods. This is largely attributed to its greedy nature. Other decision-tree algorithms overcome this issue by generating a large number of trees and selecting the best performing one. The method of *random forests* produces an ensemble of CART trees (known as forest) and arrives at predictions by averaging over the predictions of each of the generated trees in the forest [10]. When each tree is generated by using a different bootstrap sample from the training data, the variance of the forest can be increased by ensuring that the splits at each stage can only be selected randomly amongst the features. A practical aspect is that each tree in the forest can be trained independently, allowing for an embarrassingly parallel computation.

2.3.3.2 Boosted trees

Boosting also allows an ensemble of trees to be generated, however, in an iterative fashion. The method of *gradient-boosted trees* is well known for its cutting edge accuracy [11]. In each iteration, a tree is trained to fit the residuals of the current collection before being added to the collection. Its weight is calculated by minimizing the overall training error of the collection, whose prediction is given by the weighted average of the trees within the collection. Therefore, the boosting process iteratively improves the overall prediction by fitting trees that select training data points with the largest errors for the respective iteration. Currently, the method of XGBoost records amongst the highest accuracies for regression and classification problems on standard datasets, in particular due to its highly-tailored implementation [12].

2.3.4 Optimal trees

More recently, the formulation of the underlying computation of CART was advanced to a mixed-integer optimization problem, which could be solved to optimality due to their tractable reformulations [13]. As a result, these *optimal classification trees* (OCT) were able to provide practical solutions to real-sized problems with a sizable enhancement of accuracy over classical methods, such as

CART [9]. These OCTs are capable of combine the interpretability of trees with high accuracy that is guaranteed by optimality of the solution to the underlying optimization problem. In addition, the resulting trees prove to better reflect the ground truth, alleviating overfitting concerns that are raised for optimization-based approaches.

2.3.5 Neural networks

While the goal of cognitive and neuroscientists is the understanding of how the human brain functions (see e.g. [14, 15]), in data science and engineering the goal is to build useful machines to infer insights from data and potentially inform decisions. The powerful capability of the human brain to process information, learn, and adapt remains unmatched in man-made and artificial designs for speech recognition, vision, and learning. If we were able to understand and mimic some of the brain's capabilities in order to build machines that can augment and improve the human condition, many aspects of life and economy could be advanced. Of the many challenges in this quest is the sheer parallelism. The human brain is composed of approximately 10^{11} computing units, also known as *neurons*. Moreover, these units communicate with each other in a highly connected fashion. In fact, each neuron is believed to be connected to 10^4 other neurons. These connections, called *synapses*, also operate in parallel. To project this onto computers, the processing in the brain is accomplished by neurons and the memory is in the synapses between the neurons, resulting in processing and memory being distributed across the network. This architecture motivated the design of artificial neural networks to follow the paradigm of parallel processing.

This section extends the network representation that we developed previously towards graphical models to leverage the vocabulary of graph theory and its representational power. In this context, we associate variables with nodes of a graph. Correspondingly, transformations of these variables are based on instructions on how to propagate the values along the links of the graph. When these graphs also carry probabilistic information on the variables and their interconnections, then the weight computation of the neural network corresponds to a statistical problem. Examples are hidden Markov models, Kalman filters, and path analysis models, where one kind of model can be reduced to the other [2].

In graphical models, we need to distinguish between two types of graphs. In *undirected graphs*, the nodes (or variables) X_i and X_k are conditionally independent given X_j if nodes X_i and X_k are separated by X_j for any sets of nonidentical nodes. In *directed graphs*, on the other hand, we can have 'induced dependencies', i.e., two nodes that are marginally independent can turn conditionally dependent and reveal the value of a third node. In the example of two independent coin tosses X_i and X_j, each outcome is marginally independent, but they are conditionally dependent, given the value of their sum $X_k = X_i + X_j$. In directed graphs, where the paths may be directional (one way connection between nodes), the notion of independence differs from undirected graphs only when paths have two arrows arriving at the same node. In fact, the models we have discussed so far are directed graphs. Before we introduce examples of undirected graphs, we need to introduce some pre-processing and prior knowledge inclusion techniques which have the potential to sizably improve the results.

2.3.5.1 Pre-processing

Often, components of the input data can affect outcomes differently, heavily based on their range of values. A simple first step in pre-processing is *normalization.* It may be simple linear rescaling of each variable independently in order to obtain a zero mean and unit variance for the training set. Such scaling may be implemented as an initial layer of weights. However, computationally it is more efficient to pre-process the input and forego such an initial optimization of weights. Similarly, output values can be efficiently normalized during the pre-processing. It is often recommendable to translate labels of categorical variables to binary representation in order to leverage numerical transformations. In addition to these linear transformations, the dimensionality of the input space can be reduced to gain computational tractability, e.g., to overcome the curse of dimensionality. Such transformations may result in a loss of information that has to be traded off against the computational gains. While the selection of a subset of variables proves practical in many cases, optimal trade-offs are achieved by engineering new variables, also known as *features*, via tailored transformation of a combination of original variables. The method of *principal component analysis* poses a common approach to dimension reduction, where the original input space is mapped to a new space that is spun by linear combinations of a subset of the original variables [3, 16, 17]. Note that dimension reduction techniques typically do not affect the output values, which might affect the quality and reliability of the learning.

2.3.5.2 Inclusion of prior knowledge

In many real-world settings, leveraging system inherent *prior knowledge* provides additional performance improvements. For example, when the position of some information in the data is irrelevant to the classification (e.g., when recognizing handwritten digits), then this *translation invariance* can be accomplished via the *shared weights* method, where the units of the hidden layers in a network take inputs from a smaller subset of units from the previous layer. When the neighboring units are constrained to common weights, the network output becomes insensitive to translations of the input values. This redundancy by weight sharing also improves complexity by reducing the number of independent variables compared to the number of weights. Alternatively, one can inflate the training set by generating virtual samples via transformations of the original training set [18].

2.3.5.3 Example of an undirected graphical model: Boltzmann machine

A Boltzmann machine is an undirected probabilistic graph with conditionally independent nodes [19]. In general, each node can be regarded as a discrete random variable X_i and the probability distribution of the possible configurations is given by an *energy function E*, which be expressed for the configuration index α of the nodes X_i and X_j as $E_\alpha = -\sum_{i<j} J_{\mathrm{ij}} X_i^\alpha X_j^\alpha$, where J_{ij} is the symmetric weight on the link between

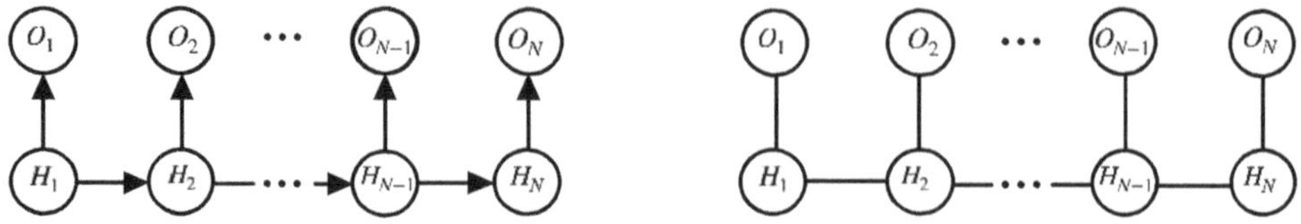

Figure 2.3. Illustration of graphical models with horizontal links as transition matrix A and vertical links as emotion matrix B along with the parameters corresponding to the logarithms of the respective matrix elements: (left) a directed graph of an HMM, and (right) an undirected graph of an HMM as a Boltzmann machine.

the nodes with $J_{ij} = J_{ji}$. Consequently, the Boltzmann distribution of the configuration α is given by the probability

$$P_\alpha = \frac{e^{-E_\alpha/T}}{\sum_\gamma e^{-E_\gamma/T}}, \tag{2.11}$$

where the scale of the energy is controlled by the *temperature* T.

2.3.5.4 Example of a directed graphical model: hidden Markov model

The hidden Markov model (HMM) is a directed probabilistic graph. It can be defined by a set of *state variables* H_i, output variables O_i, a *probability transition matrix* $A = p(H_i|H_{i-1})$, and an *emission matrix* $B = p(O_i|H_i)$ [20]. Figure 2.3(left) illustrates such a directed graph for an HMM, whereas figure 2.3(right) shows a special case of a Boltzmann machine as an HMM [21]. Under this analogy, the Boltzmann distribution of equation (2.11) transforms the energy, which has an additive nature, to a product of standard HMM probability distributions. Graphical models have the property of reducing a directed graph to an undirected graph [22].

2.3.5.5 Example of general mixture models

Similarly, general mixture models can be represented with graphical models [23]. To this end, note that the mixture density of equation (2.2) can also be viewed as a graphical model, where the two nodes consist of a multinomial *hidden node*, representing which component is selected, and a *visible node* for $\boldsymbol{x}$. These two nodes are then connected by a directed link. In the context of conditional mixture models, another visible node will be connected to both the hidden and the visible node by two directed links [24]. Subsequently, hierarchical conditional mixture models can be constructed by a chain of hidden nodes, namely a hidden node for each level of the tree [25].

2.3.5.6 Inference and learning

In the context of graphical models and neural networks, the task of inference and learning can be cast as the problem of computing the probabilities of the *hidden nodes*, given the values that were observed in other nodes, which can be regarded as *visible nodes*. In figure 2.3 for HMM, the variables O_i can be viewed as visible and the nodes H_i as hidden states. The goal is to compute the probability distribution of H_i. A similar calculation is necessary for Boltzmann machines and mixture models.

In principle, calculating the *posterior* probabilities on a graph is known to be NP-hard. Therefore, many inference algorithms focus on special cases, where this computation can be done efficiently. In the example of HMMs, their chain structure permits efficient algorithms, such as the classical forward-backward algorithm [20]. Similarly, the hierarchical structure of decision trees can be leveraged for efficient algorithms, including optimization-based methods. The described generic mixture models, Kalman filters and Boltzmann machines can also be viewed as such special cases that allow efficient computation. For graphs that do not exhibit tree or chain structures and are potentially highly connected, approximate algorithms, such as Gibbs sampling were proposed [26].

We now focus the discussion on specific designs of neural networks as they are developed in many of the current applications and are directly related to radiation therapy. To this end, note that conventional methods require careful engineering and some expertise in the underlying domain to extract suitable features that allow to transform input raw data into a representation that enables higher predictive power. More recently, the underlying representation itself has become the subject of learning.

2.3.5.7 Deep neural network

Deep-learning methods aim to learn multiple levels of representations. They are obtained by composing simple to calculate nonlinear modules, each of which transforms the representation of one layer into a representation of a higher level. Starting from the raw input values $\boldsymbol{x}$, each layer increases the level of abstraction, such that ultimately very complex functions can be learned. The architecture of a deep-learning network consists of multiple of these layers, each with the goal of improving the selectivity and the invariance of the representation. For example, in classification, higher layers of representation are capable of amplifying certain features of the input that most contribute towards separating and marginalizing irrelevant variations in the data [27]. For image recognition, the first layer typically leads to features on the presence or absence of edges at particular orientations or locations of the array of pixels of the image. The second layer then spots particular arrangements of edges, regardless of variations in edge positions, suggesting motifs. The third layer can compose motifs into extended combinations that start to resemble known objects. The subsequent layers then identify objects as combinations of such segments. Notice that these layers of deep learning are neither engineered by humans nor designed to be understandable and interpretable by humans.

Recent developments in deep learning have manifested some significant breakthroughs in many areas, from speech [28–30] and image recognition [31–33] to understanding particle accelerator data [34, 35] and drug design [36]. Some of the astonishing improvements of deep learning were reported in the area of understanding of natural languages [37], for example in answering questions [38] and translation [39].

In deep learning, the weight vectors for the learning algorithm are computed in an alternative way that provides significant speed up and does not impose dependence on the underlying probability functions. More specifically, the learning algorithm provides a gradient vector for each vector, determining the amount of error increase or decrease depending on the weight increase or decrease. Consequently, the weight vector is adjusted opposite to the gradient vector, following an iterative gradient descent.

2.3.5.8 Stochastic gradient descent

The objective function, which typically measures the learning error, can be regarded as a higher dimensional surface on the space of weight values, when it is averaged over all training samples. Consequently, the negative gradient on this surface of the current iterate indicates the direction of the steepest descent over this landscape and updating along this direction by an appropriate step size lowers the output error on average. In practice, it is more efficient to collect a few samples of the input vector and to compute the outputs and the corresponding errors before evaluating the average gradient for these samples, in order to update the weights accordingly. This method of *stochastic gradient descent* (SGD) iterates for many of these small sets of samples within the training data until the average objective function converges, i.e., no longer decreases by a sizable amount. The stochasticity stems from the errors introduced when estimating the average gradient over the samples. For a broad range of applications, this fairly simple procedure can find a good set of weights quicker, when compared to deterministic optimization algorithm [40]. In some cases, computing gradients can be challenging.

2.3.5.9 Backpropagation

Whenever the nodes are smooth functions of their inputs and their respective weights, it has been shown that the gradients can be evaluated with the *back-propagation procedure*, which in essence is the application of the chain rule of derivation [41–43]. The gradient of the objective function with respect to the input of a node is calculated by working backward from the gradient with respect to the input of the subsequent node (which is the output of the current node). The recursive procedure can be applied to propagate gradients through all nodes, starting from the output all the way backward to the input variables. Once these gradients become available, one can straightforwardly determine the gradient with respect to the weights of each node. This method offers an alternative to the feed-forward approach that we discussed earlier.

2.3.5.10 Convolutional NN

Another class of feed-forward deep-learning networks that have proved particularly successful in computer vision are the *convolutional neural networks* (CNN), which often train more efficiently and are more generalizable than networks with connectivity between neighboring layers [44]. CNNs are well suited for multi-arrayed data, such as color images composed of three two-dimensional arrays of intensity pixels, each in the three color channels of RGB. Many applications exhibit such a structure, e.g., signals and sequences such as languages can be viewed as one-dimensional, images or audio spectrograms can be cast as two-dimensional arrays, and volumetric images as three-dimensional structures. CNNs leverage four aspects to harness fundamental properties of the incoming signal, namely (i) local connections, (ii) shared weights, (iii) pooling, and (iv) the use of many layers. Depending on the type of application, these four ideas motivate the structure of the CNN with their respective importance.

A typical CNN exhibits an architecture that is composed of a series of stages [27]. The first few stages consist of two types of *convolutional* and *pooling layers*. Nodes with a convolutional layer are arranged by their feature maps. Each unit within a map is connected to local subsets in the feature maps of the previous layer. The set of weights of these links is called a *filter bank*. The weighted sum of each localized subset of features is then the argument of *rectified linear unit* (ReLU), which removes potential negative values, for example via an activation function $f(\cdot) = \max(0,\cdot)$. This procedure introduces desired nonlinearities to the network's decision function without changing the receptive fields of the layer. Within each local feature map, all nodes share the same filter bank and different feature maps within the same layer can employ different filter banks. This structure allows to leverage the high correlation amongst groups of values within a data array in order to assemble local motifs to enhance detection. Furthermore, it reflects the location invariance of local statistics of the data array. This filtering operation by a feature map can be computed by a discrete convolution, allowing for the detection of local conjunctions of features from the previous layer.

A pooling layer, on the other hand, serves to merge semantically close features into one. Here, the maximum of a local section of nodes in one feature map is computed. Then, neighboring pooling units receive input from sections that are translated by more than one column or row. This translation ensures the invariance to translation or distortions. A typical CNN architecture is composed of a few stacked stages of convolution, nonlinearity, and pooling, followed by additional convolutional and fully connected layers [27]. The backpropagating gradients can then be computed through the CNN analogous to a regular deep network by training all the weights in all the filter banks. This structure was derived from the hierarchy in the visual cortex ventral pathway [45].

2.3.5.11 ResNet and DenseNet

Since CNN architectures allow deeper networks, the accuracy can become saturated beyond a certain depth and suddenly degrade. Interestingly, this *degradation problem* is not due to overfitting. Moreover, including more layers for a sizably deep network will cause higher training errors [46]. *Residual neural network* (ResNet) model can address this degradation problem by skipping some of the connections or even jumping over several layers [47]. ResNet models contain ReLU as well as batch normalization of the weights.

To accelerate this process, several skips can be designed in parallel. These *dense convolutional network* (DenseNet) connect many layers to many other layers in a feed-forward structure. In fact, for each layer, the feature maps of all previous layers are used as an input, and its own outputs are used as inputs of all the following layers, resulting in $L(L + 1)/2$ direct connections between the L layers, whereas a conventional CNN would have only L connection [48]. A typical problem of CNNs is that in some cases the gradients do not converge because they vanish or explode [49]. DenseNet can overcome this problem by construction. Furthermore, they strengthen the feature propagation and allow feature reuse, reducing the number of parameters.

2.4 Summary

Given the broad range of applications that have witnessed success driven by artificial intelligence and machine learning, this chapter provides a unifying introduction to this field. Rather than discussing the details for specific applications, we started with the basic principles of learning that allows construction of a unifying framework for many common and currently used methodologies, in particular in the context of radiation therapy. We show the connecting bridges between mixture models, regression and classification models, decision trees, as well as neural networks. Details on how these methods are extended to different aspects of radiation therapy will be discussed in the following chapters.

2.5 Acknowledgement

We would like to thank Alessandro Previero for insightful discussions.

References

[1] Tarassenko L, Hayton P, Cerneaz N and Brady M 1995 Novelty detection for the identification of masses in mammograms *IET Conf. Proc.* 442–47

[2] Jordan M I and Bishop C 1997 ed A B Tucker *CRC Handbook of Computer Science* (Boca Raton, FL: CRC Press)

[3] Anderson T W 1984 *An Introduction to Multivariate Statistical Analysis* (New York: Wiley)

[4] Duda R O, Hart P E and Stork D G 1973 *Pattern Classification and Scene Analysis* (New York: Wiley)

[5] Bishop C M *et al* 1995 *Neural Networks for Pattern Recognition* (Oxford: Oxford University Press)

[6] Breiman L, Friedman J, Stone C J and Olshen R A 1984 *Classification and Regression Trees* (Boca Raton, FL: CRC Press)

[7] Friedman J H 1977 *A* recursive partitioning decision rule for nonparametric classification *IEEE Trans. Comput.* **26** 404–08

[8] Breiman L and Stone C 1978 *Parsimonious binary classification trees*, Technology Service Corporation, Santa Monica, Calif. Tech. Rep. TSCCSD-TN, **4**

[9] Bertsimas D and Dunn J 2019 Machine learning under a modern optimization lens *Dynamic Ideas LLC.*

[10] Breiman L 2001 Random forests *Mach. Learn.* **45** 5–32

[11] Friedman J H 2001 Greedy function approximation: a gradient boosting machine *Ann. Stat.* 1189–232

[12] Chen T and Guestrin C 2016 XGBoost: a scalable tree boosting system *Proc. of the 22nd ACM SIGKDD Int. Conf. on Knowledge Discovery and Data Mining* 785–94

[13] Bertsimas D and Dunn J 2017 Optimal classification trees *Mach. Learn.* **106** 1039–82

[14] Posner M I 1989 *Foundations of Cognitive Science* (Cambridge, MA: MIT Press)

[15] Thagard P 2005 *Mind: Introduction to Cognitive Science* (Cambridge, MA: MIT Press)

[16] Pearson K 1901 On lines and planes of closest fit to systems of points in space *Lond. Edinb. Dublin Phil.l Mag. J. Sci.* **2** 559–72
[17] Hotelling H 1933 Analysis of a complex of statistical variables into principal components *J. Educ. Psychol.* **24** 417
[18] Vetter T and Poggio T 1997 Linear object classes and image synthesis from a single example image *IEEE Trans. Pattern Anal. Mach. Intell.* **19** 733–42
[19] Hinton G E and Sejnowski T J *et al* 1986 Learning and relearning in Boltzmann machines *Parallel Distributed Processing: Explorations in the Microstructure Of Cognition* (Cambridge, MA: MIT Press) **1** 2
[20] Smyth P, Heckerman D and Jordan M I 1997 Probabilistic independence networks for hidden markov probability models *Neural Comput.* **9** 227–69
[21] Saul L K and Jordan M I 1995 Boltzmann chains and hidden Markov models *Advances in Neural Information Processing Systems (NIPS)* 435–42
[22] Jordan M I *et al* 2004 Graphical models *Statistical Science* **19** 140–55
[23] Buntine W L 1994 Operations for learning with graphical models *J. Artif. Intell. Res.* **2** 159–225
[24] Jacobs R, Jordan M, Nowlan S and Hinton G 1991 Adaptive mixtures of local experts *Neural Comput.* **3** 79–87
[25] Jordan M I and Jacobs R A 1994 Hierarchical mixtures of experts and the em algorithm *Neural Comput.* **6** 181–214
[26] Plummer M *et al* 2003 Jags: A program for analysis of Bayesian graphical models using Gibbs sampling *Proc. of the 3rd Int. Workshop on Distributed Statistical Computing (Vienna, Austria)* **124** 1–10
[27] LeCun Y, Bengio Y and Hinton G 2015 Deep learning *Nature* **521** 436–44
[28] Hinton G, Deng L, Yu D, Dahl G E, Mohamed A-R, Jaitly N, Senior A, Vanhoucke V, Nguyen P and Sainath T N *et al* 2012 Deep neural networks for acoustic modeling in speech recognition: the shared views of four research groups *IEEE Signal Process Mag.* **29** 82–97
[29] Mikolov T, Deoras A, Povey D, Burget L and Cernocky J 2011 Strategies for training large scale neural network language models *2011 IEEE Workshop on Automatic Speech Recognition and Understanding* (Piscataway, NJ: IEEE) 196–201
[30] Sainath T N, Mohamed A-r, Kingsbury B and Ramabhadran B 2013 Deep convolutional neural networks for LVCSR *2013 IEEE Int. Conf. on Acoustics, Speech And Signal Processing* (Piscataway, NJ: IEEE) 8614–618
[31] Krizhevsky A, Sutskever I and Hinton G E 2012 Imagenet classification with deep convolutional neural networks *Adv Neural Inf Process Syst.* **25** 1097–105
[32] Farabet C, Couprie C, Najman L and LeCun Y 2012 Learning hierarchical features for scene labeling *IEEE Trans. Pattern Anal. Mach. Intell.* **35** 1915–29
[33] Tompson J, Jain A, LeCun Y and Bregler C 2014 Joint training of a convolutional network and a graphical model for human pose estimation *arXiv preprint arXiv* 1406.2984
[34] Adam-Bourdarios C, Cowan G, Germain C, Guyon I, Kegl B and Rousseau D *et al* 2015 The Higgs boson machine learning challenge *NIPS 2014 Workshop on Highenergy Physics and Machine Learning,* (PMLR) 19–55
[35] Ciodaro T, Deva D, De Seixas J and Damazio D 2012 Online particle detection with neural networks based on topological calorimetry information *J. Phys.: Conf. Ser.* 368 012030
[36] Ma J, Sheridan R P, Liaw A, Dahl G E and Svetnik V 2015 Deep neural nets as a method for quantitative structure–activity relationships *J. Chem. Inf. Model.* **55** 263–74

[37] Collobert R, Weston J, Bottou L, Karlen M, Kavukcuoglu K and Kuksa P 2011 Natural language processing (almost) from scratch *J. Mach. Learn. Res.* **12** 2493–537
[38] Bordes A, Chopra S and Weston J 2014 Question answering with subgraph embeddings arXiv **1406** 3676
[39] Sutskever I, Vinyals O and Le Q V 2014 Sequence to sequence learning with neural networks *Proc. Advances in Natural Information Processing Systems* **27** 3104–12
[40] Bottou L and Bousquet O 2011 The tradeoffs of large-scale learning *Optimization for Machine Learning* 351
[41] Werbos P 1974 Beyond regression: new tools for prediction and analysis in the behavioral sciences *PhD Thesis* Harvard University
[42] Parker D B 1985 *Learning Logic* Report TR-47 (Cambridge, MA: MIT Press)
[43] Rumelhart D E, Hinton G E and Williams R J 1986 Learning representations by backpropagating errors *Nature* **323** 533–36
[44] LeCun Y, Boser B and Denker J 1989 Handwritten digit recognition with a backpropagation network *Proc. Advances in Neural Information Processing Systems* 396–404
[45] Felleman D J and Van Essen D C 1991 Distributed hierarchical processing in the primate cerebral cortex *Cereb. Cortex* **1** 1–47
[46] He K and Sun J 2015 Convolutional neural networks at constrained time cost *Proc. of the IEEE Conf. on Computer Vision and Pattern Recognition* 5353–60
[47] He K, Zhang X, Ren S and Sun J 2016 Deep residual learning for image recognition *Proc. of the IEEE Conf. on Computer Vision and Pattern Recognition* 770–78
[48] Huang G, Liu Z, Van Der Maaten L and Weinberger K Q 2017 Densely connected convolutional networks *Proc. of the IEEE Conf. on Computer Vision and Pattern Recognition* 4700–708
[49] Bengio Y, Simard P and Frasconi P 1994 Learning long-term dependencies with gradient descent is difficult *IEEE Trans. Neural Networks* **5** 157–66

Chapter 3

Overview of AI applications in radiation therapy

Yang Sheng and Jiahan Zhang

Artificial intelligence has seen substantial progress in modern radiation therapy in recent years thanks to the improvement of computational power and the increasing availability of data. This chapter will break down details of technological advancement in various steps in a routine radiation therapy workflow, starting from diagnosis, simulation, to treatment planning, delivery and assessment. Researchers employ powerful machine learning algorithms to aim for more accurate target delineation, faster treatment planning, safer treatment delivery and better treatment outcome. Contributions from researchers over the years has resulted in AI being used in busy radiation oncology departments and more application is expected in the near future.

3.1 Opportunities of AI applications in modern radiotherapy workflow

Radiation therapy aims to deliver a highly conformal dose to the entire tumor while trying to minimize the radiation damage to the surrounding healthy tissue. The traditional radiation therapy workflow is, from start to finish: patient assessment, anatomy acquisition via simulation imaging, target and organs-at-risk (OARs) delineation, treatment prescription, treatment planning, quality assurance, setup verification, treatment delivery and treatment follow-up/assessment (figure 3.1). A successful radiation therapy program relies heavily on a high standard of equipment as well as well-trained team members. Several key steps in radiation therapy workflow need substantial training and experience from the staff to deliver high quality services. Such a process could take years and is heavily resource demanding. In addition, the lack of training and experience could yield a subpar quality of service and could potentially jeopardize the treatment outcome.

Radiation therapy has been a highly standardized discipline and yet innovative. With the advent of more powerful computation power, machine learning and artificial intelligence (AI) saw increasing interest in radiation therapy application.

doi:10.1088/978-0-7503-3339-9ch3

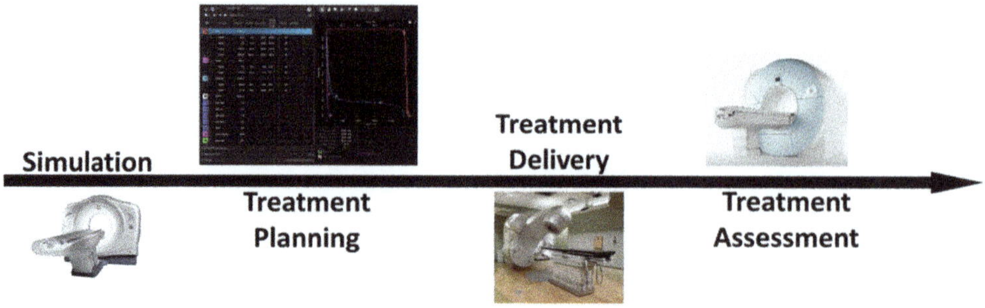

Figure 3.1. Radiation therapy workflow.

The adoption of AI in radiation therapy focuses on several key highlights, including improved workflow efficiency, customized decision-making support for patients, reduced cost and more importantly improved quality and safety for patients. AI has benefited a wide spectrum of team members in a standard radiation therapy department, including clinicians, physicists and dosimetrists. This chapter will break down several AI applications developed so far in radiation therapy workflow. We will focus on six aspects of radiation therapy workflow, including 'patient assessment', 'simulation', 'treatment planning', 'quality assurance', 'treatment delivery' and 'outcome assessment'.

(a) Patient Assessment

(i) Patient Selection

Every patient is different. Customizing the treatment for a specific patient given the metadata of the patient as well as the clinical condition is critical for a successful treatment outcome. The choice could be surgery, chemotherapy, radiation therapy or any combination of those. Building AI models utilizing clinical indicators from previous cases can help the decision-making process and improving the chance of treatment success.

Utilizing imaging features has been the main stream in assisting decision making of treatment choice. The advancement of imaging techniques has enabled early detection as well as more accurate staging for metastatic diseases. Kann *et al* developed a deep learning convolutional neural network that is capable of accurately identifying nodal metastasis of head-and-neck (HN) cancer prior to treatment [1]. A 3D convolutional neural network was trained using CT dataset with segmented lymph node samples. The proposed model was able to achieve an area under the receiver operating characteristic curve (AUC) of 0.91. Another effort has been reported by Ibragimov *et al* to predict liver stereotactic body radiation therapy (SBRT) outcomes [2]. They developed a multi-path neural network utilizing dose information, patient demographic information and anatomical information etc to directly predict post-treatment survival rates and local cancer progression. The developed AI model was able to achieve superior performance than the benchmark support vector machine and random forest models. The proposed model could effectively filter liver cancer patients who are suited to receiving SBRT treatment with promising outcomes. A similar effort in selecting a treatment regimen has been reported by Oberije *et al* [3] A stratified Cox regression model was developed to predict the overall survival for stage III non-small cell lung cancer patient receiving radiation therapy. Such decision support system could provide valuable information in customizing treatment scheme for individual patients.

(ii) Prescription

Radiation therapy dose prescription has been a highly standardized routine practice. Without substantiated clinical evidence, navigating away from widely accepted dose prescription faces tremendous risks. Novel clinical trials using an accelerated treatment regimen, or SBRT/SRS, has attracted interest in recent decades thanks to more accurate target delineation, online localization accuracy and delivery accuracy. Yet, prescribing the radiation therapy based upon basic clinical features such as tumor imaging features, lab test etc has been the routine. A novel endeavor in customizing radiation therapy dose has been reported by Lou *et al* [4]. They developed a deep neural network using pre-radiation-therapy CT and associated radiomics features to predict potential treatment failure which could then be used to guide individualized radiation therapy dose prescription. This novel approach has never been reported before and could potentially reformat the way radiation oncologists determine and prescribe radiation treatment. Some other efforts in using AI to customize the dose have been reported. Murrell *et al* [5] discussed a decision-making model for ultra-central lung tumor treatment whether the target coverage or the OAR sparing should be prioritized. This decision support model is assisted with a radiobiological model to balance the local control and OAR toxicity where they found 60 Gy in eight fractions is the optimal solution to maximize the control while maintaining acceptable dose to OAR. Allibhai *et al* [6] developed a decision support system for inoperable early stage non-small cell lung cancer. They answered the question whether a large primary tumor could potentially compromise the treatment outcome of lung SBRT which is traditionally known for small-volume tumors.

(b) Simulation

(i) Technical Selection

Simulation has been one of the key components in modern radiation therapy workflow. Acquiring patient anatomical information using various imaging modalities could provide clinicians with invaluable information for accurate staging and gross tumor delineation. A modern CT simulator has become standard equipment for a radiation oncology department. Depending on the treatment site, the CT imaging protocol could vary to maximize the visualization of the anatomy. CT simulation serves the fundamental purpose of acquiring patient anatomy to proceed with virtual simulation and planning. However, for certain anatomical sites, such as abdominal and cranial lesions, CT is not the ideal candidate to provide biological information due to limited soft tissue contrast. With technological development in recent years, the MR simulator has become a supplemental simulation equipment. An MR simulator could provide superior soft tissue contrast, important specifically for cranial radiosurgery, abdominal diseases etc. Fusing MR images to simulation CT has become the routine practice for a radiosurgery department. Other imaging modalities such as positron emission tomography (PET) has also gained interest. PET provides metabolic information of high glucose consuming cells within the body, which are highly suspected as cancerous cells. PET has become a standard imaging modality in a radiology department to detect metastatic disease in order to more accurately determine the disease staging. Yet, oncology departments are not widely equipped with PET. The availability of PET imaging could help more accurately delineate nodal disease involvement such as those commonly seen in head-and-neck cancer [7] and gastrointestinal cancer [8]. These two sites typically see substantial anatomical changes during the course of radiation therapy and therefore PET has gained utility in adaptive radiation therapy. Metabolic functionality information during the course of the treatment could help determine the treatment response and, therefore, adapt the treatment volume delineation.

The uniqueness of CT simulation in a radiation oncology department versus a radiology department comes in several aspects. First, the fundamental purpose of acquiring CT in a radiation therapy workflow is to acquire a snapshot of the patient anatomy and subsequently use it for treatment planning purposes. Anatomy reproducibility is of supreme importance in the radiation therapy workflow. Therefore, a routine CT simulator adopts a carbon fiber flat top couch which matches that on a medical linear accelerator. In contrast, the diagnostic CT often uses a curved surface couch top. Secondly, in order to establish the coordinate system for treatment planning purposes, a laser system is employed in the CT simulator to establish 'CT zero', which will be the basis for online patient alignment prior to initiating the treatment. Last but not least, the respiratory tracking system, like the real-time position management (RPM) system used by Varian Medical Systems (Palo Alto, CA, USA), is routinely used to track the breathing motion in real time.

Treatment sites such as lung, liver and upper abdomen disease enjoy the assistance of a respiratory tracking system to help accurately deliver radiation dose in real time. In recent years, more advanced technologies in AI have invested in respiratory tracking to reduce potential breathing irregularity, delays in response etc.

The challenge of respiratory gating/tracking mainly lies in breathing irregularity and delay in response. One popular solution to these dilemmas is to predict the respiratory motion in real time. Krauss *et al* evaluated the benchmark performance of various respiratory motion prediction algorithms, including linear regression, neural network, kernel density estimation and support vector regression [9]. Tatinati *et al* developed an ensemble framework to predict breathing motion for adaptive radiotherapy [10]. They adopted a stacked regression ensemble framework to exploit a low-level learner which will generalize well for the testing cases. The result showed significant improvement relative to previously reported methods. Lin *et al* further expands the respiratory motion prediction using a deep neural network [11]. They developed a long short-term memory based generalized model for prediction which outperforms conventional neural network model.

(ii) Image Acquisition

CT imaging protocols for radiation therapy treatment planning purposes have been well-established. Supplemental imaging information could assist a clinician's decision making, simplify the treatment planning workflow and improve overall safety. Recent years have seen increased use of MR simulator in radiation oncology departments to provide complementary anatomical and functional information to CT simulation. The current standard still requires CT simulation to be done to provide accurate anatomy representation and electron density information for accurate dose calculation. The superior soft tissue contrast has motivated researchers to investigate the possibility of MR-only simulation workflow. The challenges of MR-only workflow lie upon the fact that MR signal does not provide electron density information which is critical for dose calculation.

Several studies have investigated a MR-only radiation therapy workflow. Tyagi *et al* reported a MR-only simulation workflow using a commercially available MRCAT package for prostate treatment planning [12]. The package is capable of generating synthetic-CT from T2-weighted MR images. The results demonstrated clinically acceptable results and decent workflow efficiency. Hsu *et al* reported a methodology to generate synthetic-CT from MR scans for head-and-neck radiation therapy [13]. They utilized fuzzy c-means clustering method to differentiate tissues using T1-weighted, T2-weighted and two echoes from an ultra-short TE sequence images. The attenuation property is assigned to each pixel based on the probability of individual tissue class, which is subsequently converted to synthetic-CT. The resulting images showed similar contrast between bone and soft tissue as compared to simulation CT. A deep convolutional neural network approach was proposed by Maspero *et al* [14] and Olberg *et al* [15]. Maspero *et al* developed a conditional generative adversarial network (GAN) model to generate synthetic-CT from T1-weighted MR images for pediatric brain photon and proton radiation therapy [14]. Olberg *et al* proposed a deep spatial pyramid convolutional framework to generate synthetic-CT from MR images. The results showed improved performance as compared to well-established convolution GAN model. The aforementioned advancement in MR-only workflow showed promising future direction of simplified workflow while incorporating superior visualization of soft tissue contrast in radiation therapy treatment planning.

(c) Treatment Planning

(i) Image Segmentation

Radiation therapy treatment planning aims to hand-craft highly conformal radiation dose to the clinician delineated planning target volume (PTV) while minimizing radiation dose to the OARs. Successful radiation therapy treatments rely heavily on the accuracy of contour delineation. In a RTOG multi-institutional trial of normal structure delineation for breast cancer, it was found the inter-observer variability is quite substantial [16]. In addition, contour delineation/image segmentation is a time-consuming task while high accuracy is demanded. Therefore, automating the segmentation process gains substantial interest to streamline the process and improve accuracy and consistency.

Atlas-based image segmentation has been widely adopted to guide automatic segmentation. The performance of the atlas-based approach relies on the completeness of the site-specific atlas as well as the site-specific contour similarity measures. This approach has been widely implemented in commercial platforms for radiation therapy treatment planning purposes [17–24]. Another popular approach being heavily investigated in recent years is deep learning based auto-segmentation. A commercially available platform has been previously reported using U-net architecture [25–27]. The achieved contour similarity was comparable in terms of inter-observer variability for OAR and clinical target volume (CTV) for treatment site of central nervous system (CNS), head-and-neck and prostate [27]. Elguindi *et al* developed a deep learning framework to automatically segment six structures for MR-only prostate treatment planning workflow. Their methods adopt the DeepLabV3+ using transfer learning. Lin *et al* specifically target automatically delineating gross tumor volume (GTV) for nasopharyngeal carcinoma (NPC) patients [28]. They used the VoxResNet architecture trained with 3D T1-, T2-, contrast-enhanced T1-weighted, and fat-suppressed T1-weighted images. The AI assisted automatic segmentation reduced the intra- and inter-observer variation, showing promising applicability of the deep learning based AI segmentation.

(ii) Image Registration

Image registration is the process of identifying a mathematical coordinate conversion matrix between two image sets. Image registration is widely applicable in the radiation therapy workflow. Since multi-modal imaging has been made popular, registering images from different modalities has played an important role in the success of accurately identifying the treatment volume as well as aligning the patient prior to the treatment. For cranial radiosurgery, for example, SPGR+c sequence MR images are the standard protocol image sequence to delineate lesions, while the CT image serves the purpose of patient geometry definition and accurate dose calculation. Registering CT and MR images has become a routine task in a radiosurgery department. Similar application applies for abdominal treatment and spine treatment where MR provides superior soft tissue visualization.

There are two major categories of image registration. The first is rigid image registration where only the translation and rotation vectors are applied to transfer one object to the other. The distance between any two points within the object remains constant. The other category is deformable image registration (DIR), or nonrigid image registration. The distance between any two points does not necessarily remain constant, while the shape and size of the object is subject to change. In a radiation therapy context, rigid image registration often applies to cranial MR-to-CT registration and spinal MR-to-CT registration. In contrast, DIR often applies for thoracic and abdominal application, where organ motion and deformation is substantial due to breathing motion and organ peristalsis. The

American Association of Physicist in Medicine (AAPM) issued task group report No.132 discussing image registration application in radiation therapy workflow, and recommends the quality assurance approach for image registration algorithms [29]. Traditional image registration algorithms were built to maximize similarity metrics between two images. Such similarity metrics include cross correlation, mutual information, dice similarity and root mean squared error (RMSE) etc. These metrics can be defined globally or locally to balance the overall registration accuracy. Recent years have seen an increasing number of deep learning based techniques developed for image registration [30–36]. Deep neural networks excel at finding local features/landmarks which would guide image registration, even for challenging DIR tasks. Liao *et al* developed a strategy learning process to guide deep neural networks to find the best sequencing to yield the best image registration between spine CT and CBCT [32]. Wu *et al* developed a two-layer convolutional neural network to identify hierarchical representation for image patch, from which the high-level features are inferred [33]. Yang *et al* developed a fast DIR approach using a deep encoder–decoder network. It predicts momentum-parameterization of the large deformation diffeomorphic metric mapping for brain imaging [34]. Lv *et al* specifically looked at respiratory motion induced organ deformation and developed a convolution neural network-based technique to register images from different phases from the breathing cycle in MR images [36].

(iii) 3D-CRT Planning

Three-dimensional conformal radiotherapy (3D-CRT) has historically been a treatment technique and is still the workhorse in a modern radiation therapy department. 3D-CRT employs CT images to visualize a tumor target, after which the clinician drops the beam to provide adequate coverage. Navigating the beam orientation has been the key to success in 3D-CRT. Beam orientation optimization (BOO) has been heavily investigated for treatment sites such as the lung, where 3D-CRT has been predominately used. Yuan *et al* developed radiological index based method to optimize the beam angles for lung radiation therapy [37, 38]. Breedveld *et al* developed the treatment planning platform iCycle which is capable of multi-criterial beam angle optimization using a heuristic approach [39]. In addition to lung radiation therapy, beam placement for whole breast radiation therapy plays an important role in balancing breast tissue coverage and lung sparing. Wang *et al* developed a data driven approach to guide automatic beam placement for whole breast radiation therapy (WBRT) which best reflects the clinician's preference in decision making [40].

3D-CRT treatment planning aims to provide a conformal dose to the irradiated volume while balancing the beam contribution and hotspot within the volume. WBRT has been one of the most challenging treatment sites for 3D-CRT due to the irregular shape of the breast tissue. Tangential style WBRT employs either the field-in-field (FiF) technique or electronic compensation (eComp) technique provided in the Eclipse® treatment planning system by Varian Medical Systems. The FiF technique utilizes the step-and-shoot technique to equivalently deliver a modulated beam fluence. ECOMP uses the sliding window technique to deliver a modulated fluence map. ECOMP enjoys higher modulation but with the cost of more manual effort from the planner to create the optimal fluence map. Sheng *et al* developed a random forest model to automatically generate an optimal fluence map based on geometry features [41]. It is capable of reducing treatment planning time from hours to minutes. RayStation developed a more integrated automatic treatment planning module for tangential breast radiation therapy. It is powered by a heuristic optimization approach. It is capable of automatic beam placement and fluence intensity generation [42, 43].

(iv) IMRT/VMAT Planning

Intensity modulated radiation therapy (IMRT) and volumetric modulated arc therapy (VMAT) utilize a multileaf collimator (MLC) to modulate the radiation fluence that exits the Linac gantry head. Coupled with dose radiation modulation and gantry speed modulation (for VMAT), they are capable of providing a highly conformal radiation dose the target volume while nicely sparing the OAR that has never been imaginable during the 3D-CRT era. However, creating a high quality plan is not a trivial task and studies have found that the plan quality is highly dependent on the experience of the planner [44].

Initial efforts in applying machine learning and AI in automating IMRT/VMAT treatment planning focus on setting data driven planning objectives. Yuan *et al* developed the distance-to-target histogram (DTH) metric which reflects the relative geometry information between the PTV and OAR, which is the dominant factor in determining the dose spill to the OAR [45]. Principal component analysis (PCA) was employed to correlate geometric features including DTH, overlap volume percentage, in field volume percentage etc, with the output dosimetric features which are dose volume histogram (DVH) principal components (PCs). This approach achieved great success in accurately predicting DVH of OARs during inverse optimization. Varian Medical Systems introduced RapidPlan® based on this study and several validation studies have demonstrated its robustness in guiding inverse optimization [46, 47]. RapidPlan® provides the user with the capability of training a site-specific DVH prediction model to guide inverse optimization. The trained model captures the linear relation between several key aforementioned anatomical features and DVH principal components. A similar data driven approach was proposed by Wu *et al* [48]. They introduced the overlap volume histogram (OVH) to predict achievable DVH for a specific OAR. Appenzoller *et al* developed a non-parametric model to predict voxel dose as a relation with the distance to the PTV surface [49]. Other data driven approaches have focused on plan quality evaluation [50] and plan tradeoff exploration [51].

The aforementioned techniques aim to capture the OAR sparing performance based on previous training data and did not provide

PTV and OAR tradeoff information. Multi-criteria optimization (MCO) has been introduced in radiation therapy treatment planning to aid decision making without exploiting all possible solutions [52–55]. The tradeoff between the PTV and OAR constitutes the Pareto surface, where one objective cannot be improved without compromising the other. A faithful representation of the Pareto front will ask for numerous Pareto optimal plans to be generated, while this approach is not clinically feasible due to time constraints. Craft *et al* developed a linear approach to approximate the Pareto surface with finite sampling point s[53]. They found the Pareto surface is sensitive to the choice of organ objective endpoints. Craft *et al* later introduced the specific Pareto generation (PGEN) approach [55] for Pareto surface aspiration. It starts with anchor points and a single interior point, and followed by the convex hull as the upper bound approximation for the Pareto surface. The true Pareto surface will be achieved after calculating the distance from the upper bound to the lower distal point. The MCO approach provides clinicians with a valuable navigation tool to assess the tradeoff decision making for a specific patient's anatomy.

Another main stream of research direction of AI application in IMRT/VMAT treatment planning is using a deep learning approach. The aforementioned data driven approach focused on estimating achievable dose volume endpoints while not providing spatial dose information which is critical for plan evaluation. An initial effort of predicting optimal 3D dose distribution was reported by Nguyen *et al* to predict for head-and-neck radiation therapy [56] and prostate radiation therapy [57]. Later the optimal beam configuration information was incorporated into dose distribution to yield more realistic prediction [58]. Mahmood *et al* and Babier *et al* developed the 3D dose distribution prediction framework using a novel generative adversarial network (GAN) for nasopharyngeal cancer treatment [59, 60]. Converting optimal 3D dose distribution to final deliverable plan would still require inverse optimization or linear programming process. Therefore, an alternative approach using deep neural network arises to directly generate a deliverable plan. Li *et al* developed a convolutional neural network framework to predict a fluence map for prostate IMRT in real time [61]. GAN was later adopted by Li *et al* to predict a fluence map for head-and-neck radiation therapy [62]. Other challenging treatment sites such as pancreas SBRT saw success in deep learning based fluence map prediction as reported by Wang *et al* using U-net architecture [63, 64]. Ma *et al* reported an automatic fluence map generation for VMAT radiation therapy of head-and-neck [65], and this approach can be generalized to other treatment sites such as lung, liver, esophagus and prostate [66].

An alternative approach to tackling challenging treatment planning tasks is to train a versatile planning agent that is equipped with optimal planning strategy. It mimics the human learning processes of practicing, appraising reward, adapting and improving. However, it would take years of training for the human operator to gain sufficient experience. Deep reinforcement learning offers the opportunity to train an agent which interacts with the environment by simulating numerous scenarios, after which the agent reaches the optimal strategy for decision making depending the environment status. Tseng *et al* developed the deep reinforcement learning agent specifically for automatic plan adaptation for non-small cell lung cancer patients reinforcement learning [67]. Zhang *et al* trained an interpretable planning bot for pancreas SBRT, which helps humans to understand the bot better for decision making and therefore builds trust [68]. Hrinivich *et al* described a deep-Q reinforcement learning framework for machine parameter optimization based on clinical patient contour [69]. Tortora *et al* developed the deep reinforcement learning methodology for non-small cell lung carcinoma by considering radiation therapy response and cell growth [70]. Shen *et al* developed an intelligent planning agent using reinforcement learning for applications such as high dose-rate (HDR) brachytherapy [71] and prostate radiation therapy [72], and incorporated the human planner's knowledge to navigate policy search for the planning agent in order to improve the training efficiency [73].

(v) Particle Therapy Planning

Charged particles present entirely different dosimetric features as compared to photon beams in tissue. Due to increased stopping power as the charged particle decelerates, the percent depth dose (PDD) curve presents a Bragg peak towards the end of the particle range. This unique feature enables charged particle therapy, for example proton therapy and carbon ion therapy, to focus on the target volumes while sparing nearby OARs. Charged particle therapy is especially advantageous in treating tumors that are adjacent to critical OARs, such as head-and-neck, and patient sensitive to OAR doses, such as pediatric patients.

AI application in particle therapy sees success in various aspects in the treatment planning process. First is output factor and dose calculation. Grewal *et al* developed a deep learning based model to predict output factor based on patient QA data in uniform scanning proton therapy [74]. They developed Gaussian process regression (GPR) and shallow neural network (SNN) using four parameters including range, modulation, field size and measured output factor. Sun *et al* developed a machine learning approach to predict monitor units for compact proton machine [75]. They implemented three algorithms including random forest, XGBoost and Cubist using over one thousand patients' output factor measurement. Wu *et al* established a workflow using U-net architecture to convert pencil beam dose calculation to Monte Carlo based dose calculation which is the gold standard for dose calculation [76]. Another stream of AI application in particle therapy is to convert the stopping power ratio from image modalities other than CT. Several studies have reported conversion of CBCT to stopping power ratio either using the projection based method [77] or deep learning based method [78, 79], and conversion of MR to stopping power ratio [79]. Finally, knowledge-based planning also saw success in intensity modulated proton therapy (IMPT). Hall *et al* developed a predictive model for dosimetric benefit of proton therapy for skull-based tumors [80]. The model predicts OAR DVH and is trained by exploiting the correlation between the dose and the distance to the target for six OARs. Delaney *et al* reported the benchmark performance of a commercially available knowledge-based module for IMPT from Varian Medical Systems, the RapidPlanPT, which is a derivative from the photon beam counterpart RapidPlan [81]. They found comparable or improved OAR sparing while inferior dose distribution is also noticed in knowledge-based plans.

(d) Quality Assurance

Due to the complexity of the modern radiotherapy treatment planning and delivery process and the critical importance of patient safety, quality assurance (QA) has become an integral component of the radiation treatment workflow. The broader sense of QA consists of plan check and IMRT/VMAT QA. Currently, chart check tasks are typically performed manually by physicists and take substantial human efforts. This approach is repetitive and time-consuming but not as effective as automated ones. Although numerous automated or semi-automated chart check tools have been proposed in the recent years [82–85], these tools are mostly rule-based and can have varying results in different clinical environments. Alternatively, Shumway *et al* [86] took another approach and used a majority voting model, consisting of kNN, neural network, decision tree, random forest, and Adaboost, to predict the difficulty of plan check tasks. The difficult prediction system can aid the current chart checking workflow by directing more human attention to the more challenging charts and potentially increases the chance of catching planning irregularities and preventing treatment errors. With continued standardization efforts, increasingly available incident learning system data, and further developments in the field of natural language processing, it is expected that machine learning will play a larger role in the automation of the chart checking process and contribute to improved patient treatment safety.

Patient-specific IMRT/VMAT QA is another component of the pre-treatment QA process. The main purpose of IMRT/VMAT QA is to verify that the treatment plans are deliverable on the machine and identify potential discrepancies between calculated and delivered plans. The majority of patient-specific QAs are performed on the treatment machine and analyzed by physicists. Machine learning models have been developed to predict QA results in the recent years. Valdes *et al* [87, 88] implemented a Poisson Lasso regression method to predict VMAT QA passing rates with a set of handcrafted features. With this approach, Gamma passing rates for 3%/3 mm can be predicted within 3% accuracy. The metrics found to correlate well with QA results are MU per Gray, small aperture score, irregularity factor, and fraction of the plan delivered at the corners of a larger field. Li *et al* [89] compared the Poisson Lasso model with a random forest model and found that the random forest model was a better fit for QA purposes due to its improved performance in sensitivity. While the previous models rely on features handcrafted by experts with domain knowledge, recent deep learning models are capable of learning to identify potential issues regarding QA. A study by Interian *et al* [90] shows that deep neural nets with calculated fluence as input can predict QA passing rates similarly well, compared to the previous Poisson regression model, without expert supervision. More recently, Huang *et al* [91] successfully applied U-Net architecture on IMRT portal QA and accurately predicted gamma passing rates for various gamma criteria.

(e) Treatment Delivery

(i) Image Guidance

To ensure safe and effective radiation treatments, it is crucial to position the patient according to the treatment plan and align the target volumes accurately. On-board imaging techniques, such as 2D kV and CBCT, have become the standard of practice for routine patient setup. In particular, CBCT images provide 3D spatial information with the patient in the treatment position on the treatment machine and are instrumental to the success of high precision treatments such as SRS and SBRT. However, CBCT images often suffer from various artifacts due to lack of scatter rejection methods and high x-ray absorption with high-Z materials on the beam path. Various machine learning techniques have been proposed to conduct post reconstruction processing to improve CBCT image quality and address its limitations, such as reducing 4D CBCT image artifacts caused by the limited number of projections [92].

While CBCT images offer good 3D spatial information to align patients, it does not offer good soft tissue contrast. To address this problem, synthetic MR from CBCT images has been proposed to generate MR images from CBCT images [93]. In this work, the synthetic MR images are subsequently used to generate contours using an auto-segmentation module and have been shown to be superior, compared with the original CBCT images, for auto-segmentation purposes. With the community moving closer and closer toward online adaptive therapy, one major challenge that needs to be resolved is dose calculation from Linac-based imaging. On-board imaging modalities (CBCT, MV-CBCT, MR) do not offer good mapping to electron density information directly. Recently, cycle-consistent adversarial network (CycleGAN) and its variants have been applied to create synthetic CTs from CBCT [94, 95], MV-CBCT [96], and MR [97]. With synthetic-CT, it is possible to derive electron density distribution and generate accurate dose calculations. This type of information can directly address future online adaptive planning needs.

Post reconstruction processing is ultimately limited by the initial reconstruction images, and caution needs to be taken when using prior information on CBCT images, as nonexistent objects can be 'transferred' to the current patient inadvertently, which may cause errors in patient setup and tumor localization. To further improve CBCT image quality and reduce the risk of errors related to image synthesis, learning based end-to-end CBCT reconstruction methods have been proposed to learn the reconstruction process from scratch [98, 99]. With deep learning methods, high quality reconstructions can be achieved with lower CT dose or less projection data [98]. This may translate to faster image acquisition and reduction in motion artifacts.

(ii) Motion Management

With proper setup image guidance, the patient undergoing treatment can be set up to match the planned position. However, during the treatment delivery time, intra-fraction motion can still occur. To reduce such intra-fraction positioning uncertainties, numerous motion management technologies have been developed, including external marker box tracking, surface tracking, tumor marker/markerless tracking. When the target volume moves substantially within breathing cycles, breath-hold and respiratory gating are typically used to limit the size of PTV and to better spare healthy tissues from unintended high radiation dose. For patients who cannot hold breath consistently, respiratory gated treatments offer a similar level of tumor motion control. During gated treatments, beams are turned on and off based on external or internal marker positions. The most used gated treatments are based on patient breathing curves. For gated treatments, to compensate for machine response time and increase treatment delivery duty cycle, several breathing curve prediction methods have been developed. For example, Sun *et al* [100] developed an adaptive boosting and multi-layer perception (MLP) neural network-based external marker prediction method and showed that the proposed method can accurately predict 500 ms ahead of marker data acquisition. More recently, research focuses have been moved toward directly predicting tumor motions during treatment instead of predicting external markers. Lin *et al* [11] proposed a real-time respiratory motion prediction using a long short-term memory (LSTM) model. Similarly, Wang *et al* [101] developed a real-time liver tracking algorithm using LSTM with surface imaging data and demonstrated improvements over state-of-the-art supporting vector regression methods (SVR).

(f) Outcome assessment

Outcome modeling has long served the purpose of supporting clinical decision making. Early efforts on outcome predictions include handcrafted and designated features such as equivalent uniform dose (EUD), generalized equivalent uniform dose (gEUD), tumor control probability (TCP), and normal tissue complication probability (NTCP). Conventionally, statistical methods are used to correlate patient treatment outcome with such features. Bradley *et al* [102, 103] used stepwise logistic regression to predict acute esophagitis after lung treatments, and logistic regression with designed penalty function to predict pneumonitis after lung treatments. El Naqa *et al* [104] compared supporting vector machine (SVM) with linear regression for the task of predicting esophagitis, pneumonitis and xerostomia endpoints and found SVM outperformed linear regression substantially, indicating non-linear response of the endpoints with respect to the dosimetric features. Additionally, random forests [105, 106], gradient boosting machines [107], and Bayesian networks [108] have also been used to generate outcome predictions.

The current frontier of outcome modeling is to utilize learned representations from raw images and texts in patient record to directly predict treatment outcome. Zhen *et al* studied rectum toxicity prediction in cervical radiotherapy treatments with deep CNN with transfer learning [109]. In this study, VGG-16, a CNN architecture well known to the machine learning community, was used to predict patient reported toxicity grade $\geqslant 2$. The model was pre-trained using ImageNet to learn feature representations. Compared with commonly used dose volume metrics, the authors reported significantly improved prediction accuracy (AUC=0.8).

As novel deep learning based methods and traditional statistical methods continue to coexist in the field of outcome modeling, it is crucial to recognize the tradeoff of model interpretability/robustness and model expressive power. Deep learning methods are highly flexible and can be used to model complex non-linear relations between independent and dependent variables. However, it is also well documented that deep learning models sometimes pick unexpected confounding variables as features, which inevitably reduces model generalization performance. In a meta-analysis study by Isaksson *et al* [110], it has been pointed out that AUC, the most commonly used metric for evaluating model prediction accuracy, tends to be higher in smaller scale studies with less than 150 patients from a single institution. Therefore, caution should be taken when interpreting prediction accuracy results.

3.2 Summary

In recent years, researchers have developed advanced AI models to aid the radiotherapy treatment workflow and improve patient treatment safety and efficiency, from the initial patient assessment to the final treatment delivery. Many technologies discussed in this chapter have yet to reach their potential in clinics, and it will be exciting to see the technological improvements translate into clinical use in the foreseeable future. Powered by the rapid developments of modern AI concepts and the increasing ease of model deployment, novel ideas are being proposed at a pace faster than ever. Yet many challenges still remain for large scale AI model development, such as lack of high quality data and high variance in terms of clinical practice across different treatment facilities. In the meanwhile, the radiation oncology community should be aware of the risks and benefits associated with different models at different stages of the workflow before fully utilizing them clinically to avoid harming the patient inadvertently.

References

[1] Kann B H, Aneja S, Loganadane G V, Kelly J R, Smith S M and Decker R H *et al* 2018 Pretreatment identification of head and neck cancer nodal metastasis and extranodal extension using deep learning neural networks *Sci. Rep.* **8** 14036

[2] Ibragimov B, Toesca D A S, Yuan Y, Koong A C, Chang D T and Xing L 2019 Neural networks for deep radiotherapy dose analysis and prediction of liver SBRT outcomes *IEEE J Biomed Health Inform.* **23** 1821–33

[3] Oberije C, De Ruysscher D, Houben R, van de Heuvel M, Uyterlinde W and Deasy J O *et al* 2015 A validated prediction model for overall survival from stage III non-small cell lung cancer: toward survival prediction for individual patients *Int. Journal of Radiation Oncology, Biology, Physics.* **92** 935–44

[4] Lou B, Doken S, Zhuang T, Wingerter D, Gidwani M and Mistry N *et al* 2019 An image-based deep learning framework for individualising radiotherapy dose: a retrospective analysis of outcome prediction *The Lancet Digital Health.* **1** e136–47

[5] Murrell D H, Laba J M, Erickson A, Millman B, Palma D A and Louie A V 2018 Stereotactic ablative radiotherapy for ultra-central lung tumors: prioritize target coverage or organs at risk? *Radiation Oncology.* **13** 57

[6] Allibhai Z, Taremi M, Bezjak A, Brade A, Hope A J and Sun A *et al* 2013 The impact of tumor size on outcomes after stereotactic body radiation therapy for medically inoperable early-stage non-small cell lung cancer *Int. Journal of Radiation Oncology, Biology, Physics.* **87** 1064–70

[7] Krauss D J, Ye H, Yan D, Liu Q, Liang J and Marvin K *et al* 2016 Positron emission tomography (PET)–based adaptive radiation therapy for locally advanced squamous

carcinoma of the head and neck: initial results of a prospective trial *Int. Journal of Radiation Oncology, Biology, Physics.* **96** E336

[8] Bulens P, Thomas M, Deroose C M and Haustermans K 2018 PET imaging in adaptive radiotherapy of gastrointestinal tumors *Q. J. Nucl. Med. Mol. Imaging* **62** 385–403

[9] Krauss A, Nill S and Oelfke U 2011 The comparative performance of four respiratory motion predictors for real-time tumour tracking *Phys. Med. Biol.* **56** 5303–17

[10] Tatinati S, Nazarpour K, Tech Ang W and Veluvolu K C 2016 Ensemble framework based real-time respiratory motion prediction for adaptive radiotherapy applications *Med. Eng. Phys.* **38** 749–57

[11] Lin H, Shi C, Wang B, Chan M F, Tang X and Ji W 2019 Towards real-time respiratory motion prediction based on long short-term memory neural networks *Phys. Med. Biol.* **64** 085010

[12] Tyagi N, Fontenla S, Zhang J, Cloutier M, Kadbi M and Mechalakos J *et al* 2017 Dosimetric and workflow evaluation of first commercial synthetic CT software for clinical use in pelvis *Phys. Med. Biol.* **62** 2961–75

[13] Hsu S H, Cao Y, Huang K, Feng M and Balter J M 2013 Investigation of a method for generating synthetic CT models from MRI scans of the head and neck for radiation therapy *Phys. Med. Biol.* **58** 8419–35

[14] Maspero M, Bentvelzen L G, Savenije M H F, Guerreiro F, Seravalli E and Janssens G O *et al* 2020 Deep learning-based synthetic CT generation for paediatric brain MR-only photon and proton radiotherapy *Radiotherapy and Oncology: Journal of the European Society for Therapeutic Radiology and Oncology.* **153** 197–204

[15] Olberg S, Zhang H, Kennedy W R, Chun J, Rodriguez V and Zoberi I *et al* 2019 Synthetic CT reconstruction using a deep spatial pyramid convolutional framework for MR-only breast radiotherapy *Med. Phys.* **46** 4135–47

[16] Li X A, Tai A, Arthur D W, Buchholz T A, Macdonald S and Marks L B *et al* 2009 Variability of target and normal structure delineation for breast cancer radiotherapy: an RTOG multi-institutional and multiobserver study *Int. Journal of Radiation Oncology, Biology, Physics.* **73** 944–51

[17] Chaney E L, Pizer S, Joshi S, Broadhurst R, Fletcher T and Gash G *et al* 2004 Automatic male pelvis segmentation from CT images via statistically trained multi-object deformable m-rep models *Int. J. Radiat. Oncol. Biol. Phys.* **60** S153–4

[18] Grosu A-L, Lachner R, Wiedenmann N, Stärk S, Thamm R and Kneschaurek P *et al* 2003 Validation of a method for automatic image fusion (BrainLAB System) of CT data and 11C-methionine-PET data for stereotactic radiotherapy using a LINAC: first clinical experience *Int. J. Radiat. Oncol. Biol. Phys.* **56** 1450–63

[19] Commowick O, Grégoire V and Malandain G 2008 Atlas-based delineation of lymph node levels in head and neck computed tomography images *Radiother. Oncol.* **87** 281–9

[20] Hu K, Lin A, Young A, Kubicek G, Piper J W and Nelson A S *et al* 2008 Timesavings for contour generation in head and neck IMRT: multi-institutional experience with an atlas-based segmentation method *Int. J. Radiat. Oncol. Biol. Phys.* **72** S391

[21] Gooding M J, Chu K, Conibear J, Dilling T, Durrant L and Fuss M *et al* 2013 Multicenter clinical assessment of DIR atlas-based autocontouring *Int. J. Radiat. Oncol. Biol. Phys.* **87** S714–5

[22] Stewart J, Lim K, Kelly V, Xie J, Brock K K and Moseley J *et al* Automated weekly replanning for intensity-modulated radiotherapy of cervix cancer *Int. J. Radiat. Oncol. Biol. Phys.* **78** 350–8

[23] Haas B, Coradi T, Scholz M, Kunz P, Huber M and Oppitz U *et al* 2008 Automatic segmentation of thoracic and pelvic CT images for radiotherapy planning using implicit anatomic knowledge and organ-specific segmentation strategies *Phys. Med. Biol.* **53** 1751–71

[24] Sharp G, Fritscher K D, Pekar V, Peroni M, Shusharina N and Veeraraghavan H *et al* 2014 Vision 20/20: perspectives on automated image segmentation for radiotherapy *Med. Phys.* **41** 050902

[25] Wang J, Lu J, Qin G, Shen L, Sun Y and Ying H *et al* 2018 Technical note: a deep learning-based autosegmentation of rectal tumors in MR images *Med. Phys.* **45** 2560–4

[26] Nikolov S, Blackwell S, Zverovitch A, Mendes R, Livne M and De Fauw J *et al* 2018 Deep learning to achieve clinically applicable segmentation of head and neck anatomy for radiotherapy arXiv:1809.04430

[27] Wong J, Fong A, McVicar N, Smith S, Giambattista J and Wells D *et al* 2020 Comparing deep learning-based auto-segmentation of organs at risk and clinical target volumes to expert inter-observer variability in radiotherapy planning *Radiother. Oncol.* **144** 152–8

[28] Lin L, Dou Q, Jin Y M, Zhou G Q, Tang Y Q and Chen W L *et al* 2019 Deep learning for automated contouring of primary tumor volumes by MRI for nasopharyngeal carcinoma *Radiology* **291** 677–86

[29] Brock K K, Mutic S, McNutt T R, Li H and Kessler M L 2017 Use of image registration and fusion algorithms and techniques in radiotherapy: report of the AAPM Radiation Therapy Committee task group no. 132 *Med. Phys.* **44** e43–76

[30] Shan H, Jia X, Yan P, Li Y, Paganetti H and Wang G 2020 Synergizing medical imaging and radiotherapy with deep learning *Mach. Learn. Sci. Technol.* **1** 021002

[31] Sahiner B, Pezeshk A, Hadjiiski L M, Wang X, Drukker K and Cha K H *et al* 2019 Deep learning in medical imaging and radiation therapy *Med. Phys.* **46** e1–36

[32] Liao R, Miao S, Tournemire P D, Grbic S, Kamen A and Mansi T *et al* (ed) 2017 *An Artificial Agent for Robust Image Registration.* (Menlo Park, CA: AAAI)

[33] Wu G, Kim M, Wang Q, Gao Y, Liao S and Shen D 2013 Unsupervised deep feature learning for deformable registration of MR brain images *Medical Image Computing and Computer-assisted Intervention: MICCAI Int. Conf. on Medical Image Computing and Computer-Assisted Intervention.* **16** 649–56

[34] Yang X, Kwitt R, Styner M and Niethammer M 2017 Quicksilver: fast predictive image registration—a deep learning approach *NeuroImage.* **158** 378–96

[35] Miao S, Wang Z J and Liao R A 2016 CNN regression approach for real-time 2D/3D registration *IEEE Trans. Med. Imaging* **35** 1352–63

[36] Lv J, Yang M, Zhang J and Wang X 2018 Respiratory motion correction for free-breathing 3D abdominal MRI using CNN-based image registration: a feasibility study *Br. J. Radiol.* **91** 20170788

[37] Yuan L, Wu Q J, Yin F, Li Y, Sheng Y and Kelsey C R *et al* 2015 Standardized beam bouquets for lung IMRT planning *Phys. Med. Biol.* **60** 1831–43

[38] Yuan L, Zhu W, Ge Y, Jiang Y, Sheng Y and Yin F *et al* 2018 Lung IMRT planning with automatic determination of beam angle configurations *Phys. Med. Biol.* **63** 135024

[39] Breedveld S, Storchi P R M, Voet P W J and Heijmen B J M 2012 iCycle: integrated, multicriterial beam angle, and profile optimization for generation of coplanar and non-coplanar IMRT plans *Med. Phys.* **39** 951–63

[40] Wang W, Sheng Y, Yoo S, Blitzblau R C, Yin F-F and Wu Q J 2019 Goal-driven beam setting optimization for whole-breast radiation therapy *Technol. Cancer Res. Treat.* **18** 1533033819858661

[41] Sheng Y, Li T, Yoo S, Yin F-F, Blitzblau R and Horton J K *et al* 2019 Automatic planning of whole breast radiation therapy using machine learning models *Frontiers in Oncology.* **9** 750

[42] Purdie T G, Dinniwell R E, Letourneau D, Hill C and Sharpe M B 2011 Automated planning of tangential breast intensity-modulated radiotherapy using heuristic optimization *Int. J. Radiat. Oncol. Biol. Phys.* **81** 575–83

[43] Purdie T G, Dinniwell R E, Fyles A and Sharpe M B 2014 Automation and intensity modulated radiation therapy for individualized high-quality tangent breast treatment plans *Int. J. Radiat. Oncol. Biol. Phys.* **90** 688–95

[44] Nelms B E, Robinson G, Markham J, Velasco K, Boyd S and Narayan S *et al* 2012 Variation in external beam treatment plan quality: an inter-institutional study of planners and planning systems *Pract. Radiat. Oncol.* **2** 296–305

[45] Yuan L, Ge Y, Lee W, Yin F F, Kirkpatrick J and Wu Q 2012 Quantitative analysis of the factors which affect the inter-patient organ-at risk dose sparing variation in IMRT plans *Med. Phys.* **39** 6868–78

[46] Fogliata A, Belosi F, Clivio A, Navarria P, Nicolini G and Scorsetti M *et al* 2014 On the pre-clinical validation of a commercial model-based optimisation engine: application to volumetric modulated arc therapy for patients with lung or prostate cancer *Radiat. Oncol.* **113** 385–91

[47] Delaney A R, Tol J P, Dahele M, Cuijpers J, Slotman B J and Verbakel W F 2016 Effect of dosimetric outliers on the performance of a commercial knowledge-based planning solution *Int. J. Radiat. Oncol. Biol. Phys.* **94** 469–77

[48] Wu B, Ricchetti F, Sanguineti G, Kazhdan M, Simari P and Jacques R *et al* 2011 Data-driven approach to generating achievable dose-volume histogram objectives in intensity-modulated radiotherapy planning *Int. J. Radiat. Oncol. Biol. Phys.* **79** 1241–7

[49] Appenzoller L M, Michalski J M, Thorstad W L, Mutic S and Moore K L 2012 Predicting dose-volume histograms for organs-at-risk in IMRT planning *Med. Phys.* **39** 7446–61

[50] Zhang J, Wu Q J, Ge Y, Wang C, Sheng Y and Palta J *et al* 2019 Knowledge-based statistical inference method for plan quality quantification *Technol. Cancer Res. Treat.* **18** 1533033819857758

[51] Zhang J, Ge Y, Sheng Y, Wang C, Zhang J and Wu Y *et al* 2020 Knowledge-based tradeoff hyperplanes for head and neck treatment planning *Int. J. Radiat. Oncol. Biol. Phys.* **106** 1095–103

[52] Craft D, Halabi T, Shih H A and Bortfeld T 2007 An approach for practical multiobjective IMRT treatment planning *Int. J. Radiat. Oncol. Biol. Phys.* **69** 1600–7

[53] Craft D, Halabi T and Bortfeld T 2005 Exploration of tradeoffs in intensity-modulated radiotherapy *Phys. Med. Biol.* **50** 5857–68

[54] Craft D, Süss P and Bortfeld T 2007 The tradeoff between treatment plan quality and required number of monitor units in intensity-modulated radiotherapy *Int. J. Radiat. Oncol. Biol. Phys.* **67** 1596–605

[55] Craft D L, Halabi T F, Shih H A and Bortfeld T R 2006 Approximating convex pareto surfaces in multiobjective radiotherapy planning *Med. Phys.* **33** 3399–407

[56] Nguyen D, Jia X, Sher D, Lin M H, Iqbal Z and Liu H *et al* 2019 3D radiotherapy dose prediction on head and neck cancer patients with a hierarchically densely connected U-net deep learning architecture *Phys. Med. Biol.* **64** 065020

[57] Nguyen D, Long T, Jia X, Lu W, Gu X and Iqbal Z *et al* 2019 A feasibility study for predicting optimal radiation therapy dose distributions of prostate cancer patients from patient anatomy using deep learning *Sci. Rep.* **9** 1076
[58] Barragán-Montero A M, Nguyen D, Lu W, Lin M-H, Norouzi-Kandalan R and Geets X *et al* 2019 Three-dimensional dose prediction for lung IMRT patients with deep neural networks: robust learning from heterogeneous beam configurations *Med. Phys.* **46** 3679–91
[59] Mahmood R, Babier A, McNiven A, Diamant A and Chan T C Y 2018 Automated treatment planning in radiation therapy using generative adversarial networks ed D-V Finale, F Jim, J Ken, K David, R Rajesh and W Byron *et al Proc. of the 3rd Machine Learning for Healthcare Conf.; Proc. of Machine Learning Research: PMLR; J. Proc. of Machine Learning Research* 484–99
[60] Babier A, Mahmood R, McNiven A L, Diamant A and Chan T C Y 2020 Knowledge-based automated planning with three-dimensional generative adversarial networks **47** 297–306
[61] Li X, Zhang J, Sheng Y, Chang Y, Yin F F and Ge Y *et al* 2020 Automatic IMRT planning via static field fluence prediction (AIP-SFFP): a deep learning algorithm for real-time prostate treatment planning *Phys. Med. Biol.* **65** 175014
[62] Li X, Wang C, Sheng Y, Zhang J, Wang W and Yin F F *et al* 2021 An artificial intelligence-driven agent for real-time head-and-neck IMRT plan generation using conditional generative adversarial network (cGAN) *Med. Phys.* **48** 2714–23
[63] Wang W, Sheng Y, Wang C, Zhang J, Li X and Palta M *et al* 2020 Fluence map prediction using deep learning models—direct plan generation for pancreas stereotactic body radiation therapy *Frontiers in Artificial Intelligence.* **3** 68
[64] Wang W, Sheng Y, Palta M, Czito B, Willett C and Hito M *et al* 2021 Deep learning-based fluence map prediction for pancreas stereotactic body radiation therapy with simultaneous integrated boost *Adv Radiat Oncol.* **6** 10672
[65] Ma L, Chen M, Gu X and Lu W 2020 Deep learning-based inverse mapping for fluence map prediction *Phys. Med. Biol.*
[66] Ma L, Chen M, Gu X and Lu W J 2021 Generalizability of deep learning based fluence map prediction as an inverse planning approach arXiv:2104.15032
[67] Tseng H H, Luo Y, Cui S, Chien J T, Ten Haken R K and Naqa I E 2017 Deep reinforcement learning for automated radiation adaptation in lung cancer *Med. Phys.* **44** 6690–705
[68] Zhang J, Wang C, Sheng Y, Palta M, Czito B and Willett C *et al* 2020 An interpretable planning bot for pancreas stereotactic body radiation therapy *Int. J. Radiat. Oncol. Biol Phys.*
[69] Hrinivich W T and Lee J 2020 Artificial intelligence-based radiotherapy machine parameter optimization using reinforcement learning *Med. Phys.* **47** 6140–50
[70] Tortora M, Cordelli E, Sicilia R, Miele M, Matteucci P and Iannello G *et al* 2021 Deep reinforcement learning for fractionated radiotherapy in non-small cell lung carcinoma *Artif. Intell. Med.* **119** 102137
[71] Shen C, Gonzalez Y, Klages P, Qin N, Jung H and Chen L *et al* 2019 Intelligent inverse treatment planning via deep reinforcement learning, a proof-of-principle study in high dose-rate brachytherapy for cervical cancer *Phys. Med. Biol.* **64** 115013
[72] Shen C, Chen L and Jia X 2021 A hierarchical deep reinforcement learning framework for intelligent automatic treatment planning of prostate cancer intensity modulated radiation therapy *Phys. Med. Biol.* **66** 134002

[73] Shen C, Chen L, Gonzalez Y and Jia X 2021 Improving efficiency of training a virtual treatment planner network via knowledge-guided deep reinforcement learning for intelligent automatic treatment planning of radiotherapy *Med. Phys.* **48** 1909–20

[74] Grewal H S, Chacko M S, Ahmad S and Jin H 2020 Prediction of the output factor using machine and deep learning approach in uniform scanning proton therapy *J. Appl. Clin. Med. Phys.* **21** 128–34

[75] Sun B, Lam D, Yang D, Grantham K, Zhang T and Mutic S *et al* 2018 A machine learning approach to the accurate prediction of monitor units for a compact proton machine *Med. Phys.* **45** 2243–51

[76] Wu C, Nguyen D, Xing Y, Montero A B, Schuemann J and Shang H *et al* 2021 Improving proton dose calculation accuracy by using deep learning *Mach. Learn. Sci. Technol.* **2** 015017

[77] Park Y-K, Sharp G C, Phillips J and Winey B A 2015 Proton dose calculation on scatter-corrected CBCT image: feasibility study for adaptive proton therapy *Med. Phys.* **42** 4449–59

[78] Harms J, Lei Y, Wang T, McDonald M, Ghavidel B and Stokes W *et al* 2020 Cone-beam CT-derived relative stopping power map generation via deep learning for proton radiotherapy. *Med. Phys.* **47** 4416–27

[79] Thummerer A, Zaffino P, Meijers A, Marmitt G G, Seco J and Steenbakkers R J H M *et al* 2020 Comparison of CBCT based synthetic CT methods suitable for proton dose calculations in adaptive proton therapy *Phys. Med. Biol.* **65** 095002

[80] Hall D C, Trofimov A V, Winey B A, Liebsch N J and Paganetti H 2017 Predicting patient-specific dosimetric benefits of proton therapy for skull-base tumors using a geometric knowledge-based method *Int. J. Radiat. Oncol. Biol. Phys.* **97** 1087–94

[81] Delaney A R, Dong L, Mascia A, Zou W, Zhang Y and Yin L *et al* 2018 Automated knowledge-based intensity-modulated proton planning: an int. multicenter benchmarking study *Cancers* **10** 420

[82] Li H H, Wu Y, Yang D and Mutic S 2014 Software tool for physics chart checks *Prac. Radiat. Oncol.* **4** e217–25

[83] Halabi T and Lu H-M 2014 Automating checks of plan check automation *J. Appl. Clin. Med. Phys.* **15** 1–8

[84] Olsen L A, Robinson C G, He G R, Wooten H O, Yaddanapudi S and Mutic S *et al* 2014 Automated radiation therapy treatment plan workflow using a commercial application programming interface *Prac. Radiat. Oncol.* **4** 358–67

[85] Dewhurst J M, Lowe M, Hardy M J, Boylan C J, Whitehurst P and Rowbottom C G 2015 AutoLock: a semiautomated system for radiotherapy treatment plan quality control *J. Appl. Clin. Med. Phys.* **16** 339–50

[86] Shumway J W, Pillai M, Dooley J, Das S K and Chera B S 2020 Machine learning to improve the prioritization and effectiveness of pre-treatment physics chart checks *Int. J. Radiat. Oncol. Biol. Phys.* **108** S54–S5

[87] Valdes G, Scheuermann R, Hung C Y, Olszanski A, Bellerive M and Solberg T D 2016 A mathematical framework for virtual IMRT QA using machine learning *Med. Phys.* **43** 4323–34

[88] Valdes G, Chan M F, Lim S B, Scheuermann R, Deasy J O and Solberg T D I M R T 2017 QA using machine learning: a multi-institutional validation *J. Appl. Clin. Med. Phys.* **18** 279–84

[89] Li J, Wang L, Zhang X, Liu L, Li J and Chan M F *et al* 2019 Machine learning for patient-specific quality assurance of VMAT: prediction and classification accuracy *J. Radiat. Oncol. Biol. Phys.* **105** 893–902
[90] Interian Y, Rideout V, Kearney V P, Gennatas E, Morin O and Cheung J *et al* 2018 Deep nets vs expert designed features in medical physics: an IMRT QA case study *Med. Phys.* **45** 2672–80
[91] Huang Y, Pi Y, Ma K, Miao X, Fu S and Chen H *et al* 2021 Virtual patient-specific quality assurance of IMRT using UNet++: classification, gamma passing rates prediction, and dose difference prediction *Front. Oncol.* **11** 700343
[92] Madesta F, Sentker T, Gauer T and Werner R 2020 Self-contained deep learning-based boosting of 4D cone-beam CT reconstruction *Med. Phys.* **47** 5619–31
[93] Lei Y, Wang T, Tian S, Dong X, Jani A B and Schuster D *et al* 2020 Male pelvic multi-organ segmentation aided by CBCT-based synthetic MRI *Phys. Med. Biol.* **65** 035013
[94] Chen L, Liang X, Shen C, Jiang S and Wang J 2020 Synthetic CT generation from CBCT images via deep learning *Med. Phys.* **47** 1115–25
[95] Dong G, Zhang C, Liang X, Deng L, Zhu Y and Zhu X *et al* 2021 A deep unsupervised learning model for artifact correction of pelvis cone-beam CT *Front. Oncol.* **11** 686875
[96] Zhao J, Chen Z, Wang J, Xia F, Peng J and Hu Y *et al* 2021 MV CBCT-based synthetic CT generation using a deep learning method for rectal cancer adaptive radiotherapy *Front. Oncol.* **11** 655325
[97] Hsu S-H, DuPre P, Peng Q and Tomé W A 2020 A technique to generate synthetic CT from MRI for abdominal radiotherapy *J. Appl. Clin. Med. Phys.* **21** 136–43
[98] Lu K, Ren L and Yin F-F 2021 A geometry-guided deep learning technique for CBCT reconstruction *Phys. Med. Biol.* **66** 15LT01
[99] Li Y and Chen G-H 2018 *Deep Learning-based Cone Beam CT Reconstruction Framework Using a Cascaded Neural Network Architecture (Conf. Presentation)* (Bellingham, WA: SPIE)
[100] Sun W Z, Jiang M Y, Ren L, Dang J, You T and Yin F F 2017 Respiratory signal prediction based on adaptive boosting and multi-layer perceptron neural network *Phys. Med. Biol.* **62** 6822–35
[101] Wang G, Li Z, Li G, Dai G, Xiao Q and Bai L *et al* 2021 Real-time liver tracking algorithm based on LSTM and SVR networks for use in surface-guided radiation therapy *Radiat. Oncol.* **16** 13
[102] Bradley J, Deasy J O, Bentzen S and El Naqa I 2004 Dosimetric correlates for acute esophagitis in patients treated with radiotherapy for lung carcinoma *Int. J. Radiat. Oncol. Biol. Phys.* **58** 1106–13
[103] Bradley J D, Hope A, El Naqa I, Apte A, Lindsay P E and Bosch W *et al* 2007 A nomogram to predict radiation pneumonitis, derived from a combined analysis of RTOG 9311 and institutional data *Int. J. Radiat. Oncol. Biol. Phys.* **69** 985–92
[104] El Naqa I, Bradley J D, Lindsay P E, Hope A J and Deasy J O 2009 Predicting radiotherapy outcomes using statistical learning techniques *Phys. Med. Biol.* **54** S9–30
[105] Deist T M, Dankers F J W M, Valdes G, Wijsman R, Hsu I-C and Oberije C *et al* 2018 Machine learning algorithms for outcome prediction in (chemo)radiotherapy: An empirical comparison of classifiers *Med. Phys.* **45** 3449–59
[106] Desbordes P, Ruan S, Modzelewski R, Pineau P, Vauclin S and Gouel P *et al* 2017 Predictive value of initial FDG-PET features for treatment response and survival in

esophageal cancer patients treated with chemo-radiation therapy using a random forest classifier *PLoS One* **12** e0173208

[107] Yakar M, Etiz D, Metintas M, Ak G and Celik O 2021 Prediction of radiation pneumonitis with machine learning in stage III lung cancer: a pilot study *Technol. Cancer Res. Treat.* **20** 15330338211016373

[108] Luo Y, Jolly S, Palma D, Lawrence T S, Tseng H H and Valdes G *et al* 2021 A situational awareness bayesian network approach for accurate and credible personalized adaptive radiotherapy outcomes prediction in lung cancer patients *Phys. Med.* **87** 11–23

[109] Zhen X, Chen J, Zhong Z, Hrycushko B, Zhou L and Jiang S *et al* 2017 Deep convolutional neural network with transfer learning for rectum toxicity prediction in cervical cancer radiotherapy: a feasibility study *Phys. Med. Biol.* **62** 8246–63

[110] Isaksson L J, Pepa M, Zaffaroni M, Marvaso G, Alterio D and Volpe S *et al* 2020 Machine learning-based models for prediction of toxicity outcomes in radiotherapy *Front. Oncol.* **10** 790

Chapter 4

Introduction to CT/MR simulation in radiotherapy

Iori Sumida and Noriyuki Kadoya

This chapter introduces a simulation procedure for treatment plans. Immobilization devices are used for the simulation step to fix the patient in a comfortable position. Since the treatment time should be as short as possible, an appropriate immobilization device should be used that can easily reproduce the setup. In addition to the CT image, multi-modality images such as MRI and PET images have been used for organ delineation and functional evaluation. This process requires image deformation. Neural networks contribute to all areas of image translation, image deformation, and image quality improvement, which will connect with future radiotherapy.

4.1 Simulation procedure in the radiation therapy process

A simulation procedure is usually necessary to make a treatment plan for organ delineation and dose calculation. CT scanners have been used for treatment planning for many years to see patient anatomy slice by slice, this results in viewing the organ volume in three dimensions. Since CT numbers can be correlated with the physical and electron density of the tissue, we are able to calculate absorbed dose in a patient with heterogeneity correction in lung, bone, fat, and muscle. There are two purposes for image acquisitions using a CT scanner. The first is for diagnostic purposes. A diagnostic CT scanner has a curved tabletop so that it cannot reproduce patient positions. In contrast, the radiation therapy CT scanner shown in figure 4.1 has a flat tabletop and a laser used for positioning on the wall and ceiling. Therefore, patient positions can be reproduced in the same geometry in radiation therapy conditions because there are the same treatment couches and laser lights in the radiation treatment room. To gain reproducibility of patient positions, immobilization devices are used to fix patient accurately. Figure 4.2 shows a thermoplastic mask for the head and neck of cancer patients. The red arrow denotes the intersection of laser lights to aid positioning. The radiation technologist sets the

doi:10.1088/978-0-7503-3339-9ch4

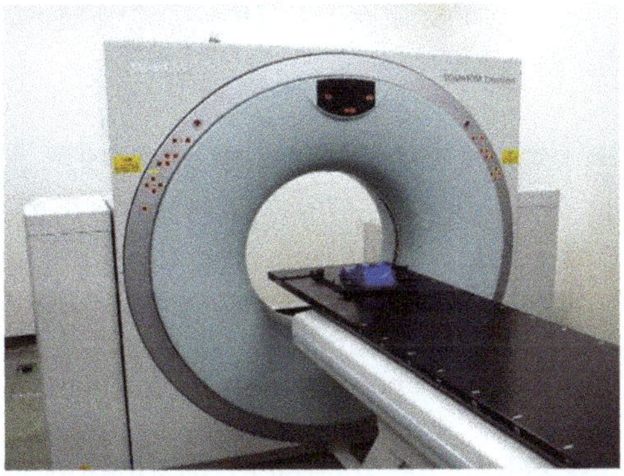

Figure 4.1. CT scanner for radiation therapy.

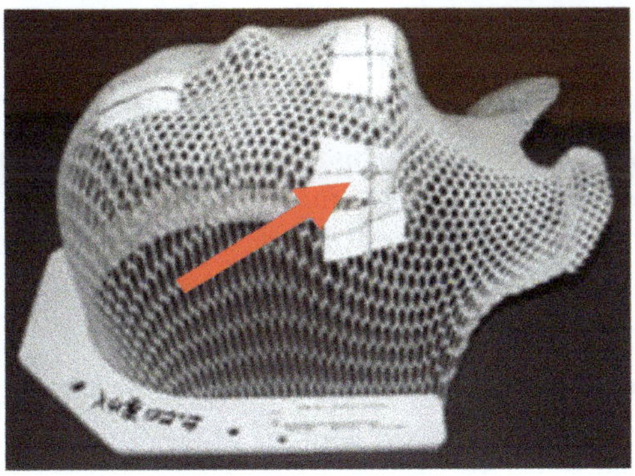

Figure 4.2. Thermoplastic mask.

intersection point on the CT scanner before taking the CT image. Then the geometry axes in the left–right, anterior–superior, and head–foot directions are defined in the patient, and the intersection point is then the origin in the DICOM coordination. Since DICOM coordination of the patient is available on the CT image, organ location on the CT image can be administrated in a treatment planning system in three dimensions.

MR scanners have been recently used for simulation purposes. Compared to a CT scan, an MR image does not show tissue density and electron density, however, it has better tissue contrast for imaging. Therefore, in radiation therapy, MRI acquisition is also used in addition to CT image acquisition. The dose calculation is performed using a CT image on the treatment planning system, and the contour drawing of the organ is posted on the CT image by fusion of the CT image and the MR image via image registration.

If there is no flat tabletop in the MR scanner, it is only used for diagnostic purposes, the patient's shape will change because of the different tabletop shapes in the radiation therapy CT scanner and the MR scanner. In that case deformable image registration (discussed later) should be adopted to mathc the MR image with the CT image. If there is an MR simulator with a flat tabletop and an MR compatible immobilization device, then an MR simulation procedure is available as well as a CT simulation procedure.

4.2 Immobilization device for radiation therapy

Three-dimensional conformal radiation therapy (3D-CRT) and intensity-modulated radiation therapy (IMRT) can deliver radiation doses to the target conformally, while sparing doses to the normal tissue. The steeper the dose gradient to the target is, the more sensitive the delivered dose to the target is due to patient position variation and organ movement. Therefore, the treatment plan developed on the treatment planning system is delivered to the patient correctly using image guidance which is performed just before the treatment irradiation to know the deviation between planned and actual locations for targeting.

The magnitude of position variation for patient setup has been investigated by many institutions. Table 4.1 shows some of these measurements and indicates a reasonable range for position variation.

It should be noted that these reported values depend on the immobilization device and procedures which are used for each treatment site. It is important that an institution determines its own position variation distributions using its own immobilization device and procedures. These distributions will then be applied as a for baseline for treatment planning and as a planning target volume margin recipe.

4.2.1 Systematic error and random error

Multiple samples of patient positions will produce a scatter distribution like that shown in figure 4.3. The distribution is generated by the image guidance at each treatment session. First, a radiation therapist sets up a patient via skin marks to isocenter. Then image acquisition is done to show the deviation between the planned and actual positions through 2D or 3D image registrations. 2D image registration is performed using digitally reconstructed radiograph (DRR) and kilovoltage or megavoltage portal images are taken via an electric portal imaging device (EPID). In contrast, 3D image registration is performed using treatment planning CT and an actual CT is taken just before treatment irradiation. Conventionally, the average coordinate of this distribution is considered as the 'systematic' error. It is the effective offset that persists throughout the samples that multiple patient positions

Table 4.1. Example measured setup variations.

Investigator	Body site	Immobilization device	Mean error (mm)	Standard deviation (mm)
Hong *et al* [1]	Head/neck	Mask and laser alignment	6.97	3.63
White *et al* [2]	Prostate	Alpha cradleHipfix	2.8	0.8
		Hipfix	5.1	1.9
Ueda *et al* [3]	Lung	Elekta body frame	3.1	3.9
Pisani *et al* [4]	Various	Not available	6.6	2.4

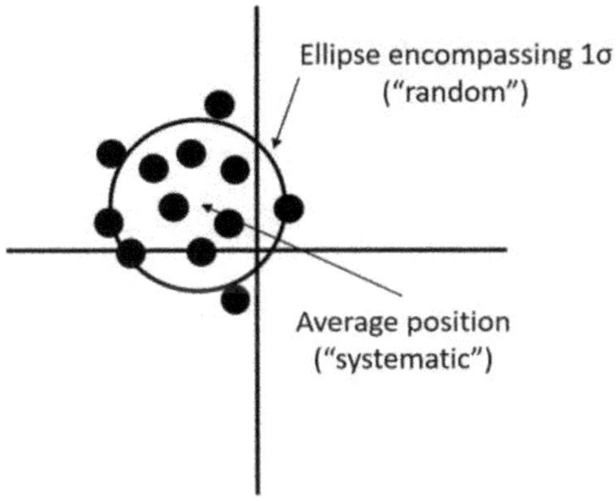

Figure 4.3. Scatter distribution of patient position over multiple samples, relative to the treatment planned position of the patient.

over a course of treatment. And the spread of sampled positions about this average coordinate represents the random setup variation.

Ideally, there should be no systematic error in patient position. However, due to discomfort caused by the immobilization device or unfamiliarity with the device and how it is used, a systematic error may be observed. Although these setup variations require wide margins to ensure target coverage in the treatment plan, which results in a dose increase to the normal tissues. Therefore, training for the preparation of immobilization devices within a department is important, so that these systematic and random errors can be reduced [5].

4.2.2 Reproducibility of patient setup

The purpose of immobilization is to limit or eliminate movement during image acquisition and radiation treatment. The main objective is to limit target motion and even the normal tissues also need to be considered. The advantage of a given immobilization method may be compromised by the complexity of use. If an immobilization device has many degrees of freedom, improper configuration of the device may lead to systematic errors in patient position or shape during treatment. Although these devices are cost effective, radiation therapist must pay close attention to use of these devices such as setup configuration per patient, and documented photograph of setup. To set up a patient accurately with reproducibility, a proper immobilization device should be used to a patient who is positioned comfortably. Because the simulation procedure takes 30 min, the patient is immobilized for the whole of that time. Simulation processes and treatment which take place in uncomfortable positions for patient will lead to systematic errors and will increase random errors .

4.3 Image quality and acquisition time

Image quality of CT depends on radiation exposure which is adjusted by tube current and exposure time. Figure 4.4 shows phantom CT images with the different radiation exposure.

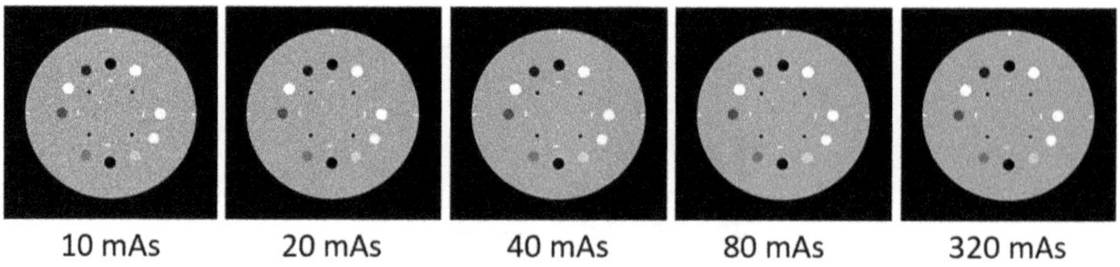

Figure 4.4. Phantom CT images with the different radiation exposure.

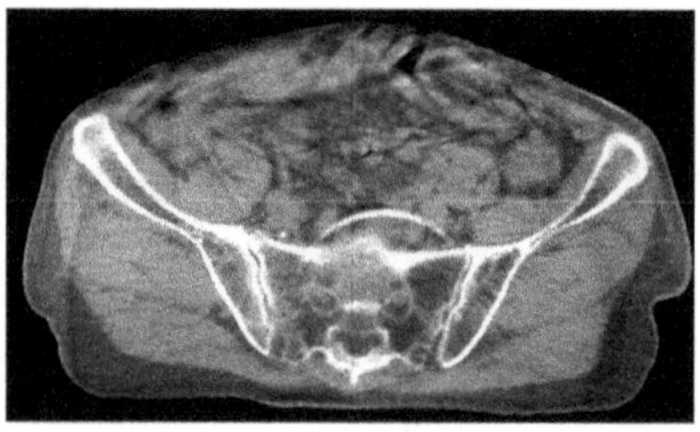

Figure 4.5. Motion artifact on CBCT image.

The photon fluence, or total number of photons at any point in the x-ray beam, is proportional to the product of the tube current and the duration of the time that the tube is firing. Therefore, increase in tube current and exposure time results in better image quality. The configuration of image acquisition is basically optimized by auto-exposure control (AEC) [6] according to the depth of the patient body obtained by a scanogram. In addition to that the radiation technologist adjusts the exposure configuration according to ALARA [7] policy.

In terms of image acquisition time, recent CT scanners rotate the x-ray tube rapidly at around 300 ms/rotation. That enables CT images to be taken from the top of the head and to the sole of the foot in a few seconds. CT images are occasionally taken under breath hold for radiation treatment plans in lung, liver, and pancreas sites, etc because the treatment planner needs to see the range of motion of the organ and this is used to decide the internal target volume (ITV). Due to the patient's condition, it might be difficult for them to hold their breath for a few seconds, in that case the radiation technologist can adjust the scan time to be as short as possible, since that leads to faster scan speed, image quality is degraded. Even when the purpose of the CT image acquisition is for organ delineation at least possible visibility, it might be allowed. Regarding cone-beam CT (CBCT) used for image guidance equipped with a linear accelerator, it takes 30 s to 1 min to acquire images. A CBCT image is reconstructed by the 2D projection image taken on EPID during gantry rotation. As such, organ motion due to breathing is projected on the EPID in 2D, that is the detector range is wider than helical CT especially in the superior–inferior direction. Therefore, this causes a motion artifact on the reconstructed image. Figure 4.5 shows a motion artifact at the anterior side of the abdomen.

4.4 Image deformation

4.4.1 Deformable image registration

As shown in figure 4.6, a deformable image registration (DIR) algorithm consists of three main parts: similarity metric (objective function), transformation model, and optimization algorithm [8, 9]. A similarity metric in DIR methods depends on how the similarity between two image sets is defined. The similarity metrics are commonly characterized into two or three categories: intensity-based (area-based or iconic), feature-based (contour-based or geometric), and combining of two similarity metrics.

The correspondences of points between two images are updated based on a transformation model. The transformation models are commonly classified into two categories: geometric (parametric) and physical (non-parametric). The geometric includes rigid, affine, free-from, global spline-based methods (e.g., thin plate splines), and local spline-based methods (e.g., B-spline). The physical contains viscous/elastic/optical flow (e.g., demons) and finite element methods (FEM). The physical models calculate transformation vectors of all points and thus require longer computation time and larger memory than the geometric models do.

The goal of the optimization is to find the best set of parameters of the transformation to obtain the best image alignment given by the similarity metric. Gradient-based methods are often used as the optimization though there are many optimization algorithms for image registration. In this section, the DIR algorithms are briefly reviewed in terms of similarity metric.

4.4.1.1 Intensity-based algorithm

An intensity-based DIR algorithm evaluates image similarity between the reference and target volumes using image intensities in an optimization problem. Mathematical methods such as the sum-of-squared differences (SSD), correlation coefficients (CC), and mutual information (MI) are used to measure the image intensity. The SSD assumes an equivalent relationship between voxel intensities in two images. Caution should be used when similar image intensities are found at many points in homogeneous regions. The intensity-based algorithm causes unrealistic image transformation in the region.

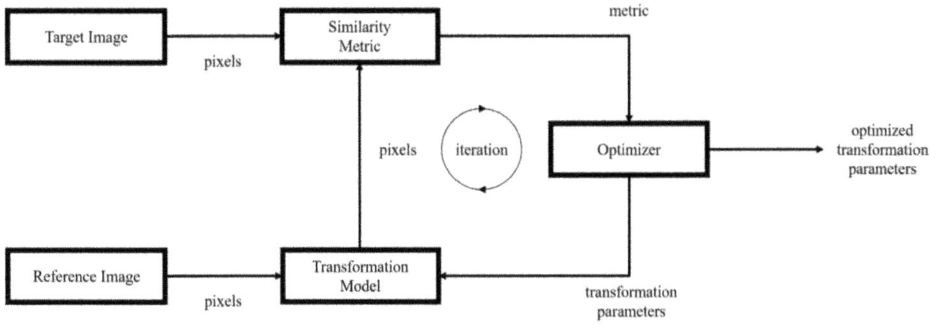

Figure 4.6. General flow chart of deformable image registration process.

The SSD is sensitive to image intensity and works well with less noisy images from the single modality such as 4D-CT data. The SSD is calculated as the average squared intensity (I_A and I_B) difference between Image A assuming reference image and Image B assuming target image, where N is the number of voxels evaluated and $I_{A'}$ is transformed Image A. The SSD is defined as equation (4.1).

$$\mathbf{SSD} = \sum_{\vec{x}} \frac{(I_B(\vec{x}) - I_{A'}(\vec{x}))^2}{N} \tag{4.1}$$

The CC between two images is less sensitive to noise in images than SSD [8]. The CC can be employed to single modality or possibly small region of multi-modality by presuming a linear relationship between voxel intensities in two images. The CC is described as equation (4.2).

$$\mathbf{CC} = \frac{\sum_{\vec{x}}(I_B(\vec{x}) - \bar{I}_B)(I_{A'}(\vec{x}) - \bar{I}_{A'})}{\sqrt{\sum_{\vec{x}}(I_B(\vec{x}) - \bar{I}_B)^2 \sum_{\vec{x}}(I_{A'}(\vec{x}) - \bar{I}_{A'})^2}} \tag{4.2}$$

where $\bar{I}_{A'}$ and $\bar{I}_B$ is the mean intensity in the Image A' and Image B, respectively. This definition is sometimes referred as zero-mean normalized cross-correlation (ZNCC). The CC is mathematically close to an inner product which is a measure that allows one to quantify how similar two mathematical objects are.

The MI is used to single or multi-modality based on an assumption on statistical relationship between voxel intensities in two images. The MI is, however, often considered the standard intensity-based objective function for DIR algorithms with multi-modality images [8]. The MI is calculated using the following equation:

$$\mathbf{MI} = \sum_B \sum_A P(I_{A'}(\vec{x}),\ I_B(\vec{x}))\log_2\left[\frac{p(I_{A'}(\vec{x}),\ I_B(\vec{x}))}{p(I_{A'}(\vec{x}))p(I_B(\vec{x}))}\right] \tag{4.3}$$

In equation (4.3), the summation is over the intensity levels in Image A' ($I_{A'}(\vec{x})$) and Image B ($I_B(\vec{x})$), where $p(I_{A'}(\vec{x}))$ and $p(I_B(\vec{x}))$ are the probability distribution functions of the intensities $I_{A'}$ and I_B, respectively. $p(I_{A'}(\vec{x}),\ I_B(\vec{x}))$ is the joint probability distribution function of the intensities at voxel occurring together.

4.4.1.2 Contour-based algorithm

A contour-based DIR algorithm which is one of the featured-based DIR algorithms (another is point-based) assumes direct relationship of identified boundaries of regions of interest in the reference and target images. Therefore, human anatomy can be taken into account. One of the advantages of the feature-based similarity metric is that the feature does not depend on the image intensity and is insensitive to noisy images such as CBCT. Thus, the contour-based DIR algorithm is applied to single or multi-modality. This algorithm is suitable for the case in which there is a contour to be registered precisely. Contours regarded as the same structure are needed to delineate on both reference and target image before the registration and this process is time-consuming. The accuracy of the delineated contours has influence on the result of the DIR. Note that similarity of the landmarks such as contours hides unrealistic image transformation in regions that are not of interest.

Surface matching is used as contour-based DIR and maximizes the overlap between corresponding surfaces extracted from two images. In the surface matching, the registration metric R is expressed as equation (4.4).

$$\boldsymbol{R} = \sum \mathbf{dist}(\boldsymbol{p}_{A'}, \boldsymbol{S}_B)^2 / \boldsymbol{N} \tag{4.4}$$

where $\mathbf{dist}(\boldsymbol{p}_{A'}, \boldsymbol{S}_B)$ calculates the minimum distance between point $\boldsymbol{p}_{A'}$ in Image A and the surfaces $\boldsymbol{S}_B$ in Image B. The summation is over the number of points, N, in Image A and the division of the summation by N is to normalize the metric.

A Chamfer matching is also used as a surface matching technique. Chamfer matching is a technique for finding the best fit of edge points from two different images, by minimizing a generalized distance between them. Chamfer matching is statistically similar to correlation. Generally, the matching problem is computation intensive however, Chamfer matching is simplified to improve computational speed. Chamfer matching segments the corresponding region in each image either automatically, often using thresholding techniques, or manually. The segmentation is then classified into an image with 0 and 1 values representing the edge of the segmented region. Minimizing the distance between the two segmented surfaces is done in the optimization.

4.4.1.3 Hybrid algorithm

A hybrid DIR algorithm is based on the intensity-based DIR algorithm combined with the feature-based technique to overcome the limitation of image-intensity-based and feature-based similarity metric. The algorithm performs the contour-based DIR in the region close to the contour and the intensity-based DIR algorithm in the region far from the contour when the contour-based DIR is adopted as the feature-based technique. As a result, more accurate deformation can be performed.

ANAtomically CONstrained Deformation Algorithm (ANACONDA) is one of the hybrid DIR algorithms and is clinically used for CT, 4D-CT and CBCT registration [10]. ANACONDA uses a CC image similarity metric, a Chamfer matching approach to minimize contour surface distances for controlling contours and grid regularization to ensure a smooth, invertible deformation. However, a CC is often used as the similarity metric and the application of the algorithm to multi-modality should be verified before clinical use.

4.4.2 AI driven image deformation

4.4.2.1 Methodologies (unsupervised, supervised learnings)

Conventional deformable image registration (DIR) techniques which were introduced in previous section have achieved high DIR accuracy in many cases, but these DIR may not be successful in the cases with poor contrast, large deformation, or multi-modality (e.g., CT-MR). In addition, these techniques require iterative calculation process, resulting in long calculation time. Although the calculation speed is improved by the GPU, the calculation time is still the bottleneck of DIR.

Therefore, to overcome these bottlenecks, AI-based DIR techniques has been developed. These techniques are roughly divided into three categories;

(1) Deep similarity metric, (2) Supervised transformation estimation, and (3) Unsupervised transformation estimation.

First, (1) deep similarity metric-based DIR is introduced. In the conventional DIR process, similarity metric, such as SSD and NCC, was used as the metric to evaluate the degree of match between fixed and deformed images in the optimization process. In this method, instead of the conventional similarity metrics, deep learning is used to learn the superior metric and generates a new deep learning-based metric. Since only the conventional similarity metric is replaced with deep learning-based metric in the conventional DIR workflow, the remining DIR process is the same as the conventional DIR process (figure 4.7). That is, the obtained is sent to the iterative optimization process, which is the same conventional process, and then the final deformation parameters (e.g., deformation vector field) and finally the deformed image is generated. In general, the learning process for deep similarity metric requires the paired annotated ground-truths (supervised learning). Cheng *et al* proposed a multi-modal stacked denoising auto-encoder based deep similarity learning method that trains a binary classifier to learn the correspondence of two image patches. The classification output was transformed to a continuous probability value, then used as the similarity score. They showed the advantage of the proposed metric for a highly accurate and robust similarity measure [11].

Next, regarding supervised transformation estimation, this method was an end-to-end method that directly estimated the DVF given a fixed and a moving image without requiring a similarity metric like conventional methods (figure 4.8). In method (1), the final transformation is estimated by the iterative optimization process, so this method cannot solve the issue of slow calculation time. On the other hand, this

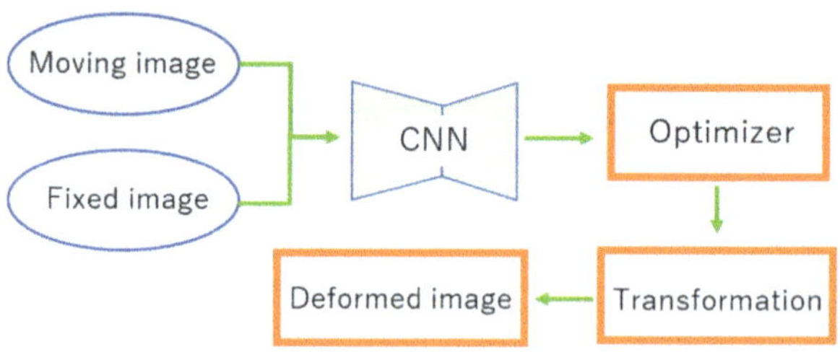

Figure 4.7. Basic framework for deformable image registration with deep similarity metric-based on the deep learning (convolutional neural network).

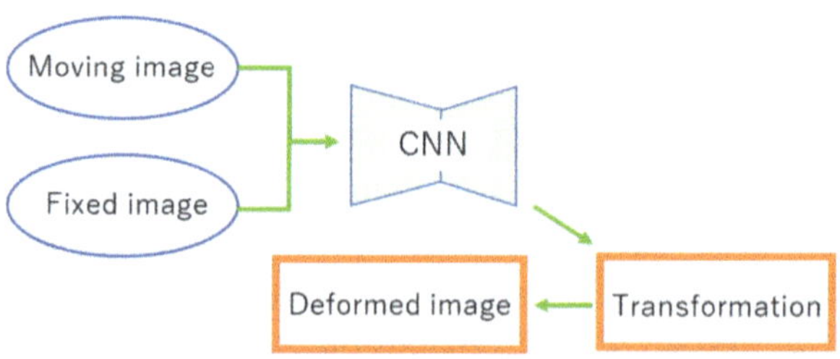

Figure 4.8. Basic framework for deformable image registration with unsupervised transformation estimation based on the deep learning (convolutional neural network).

method can solve this issue because the DVF can be estimated directly (one shot) by deep learning. Sokooti *et al* [12] proposed this method based on ResNet. This method takes patches from a pair of 3D images (fixed and moving images) as input. The output is three elements of DVF (i.e., displacement in X, Y, and Z directions) (figure 4.9). A full DVF is generated by sliding over the input images. They used two different patch sizes to incorporate local as well as more global information: $29 \times 29 \times 29$ voxel and $54 \times 54 \times 54$ voxel which are down-sampled to $27 \times 27 \times 27$ voxels. In addition, they trained the model using a large set of artificially generated DVFs. They showed that the DIR accuracy of this method was on par with a conventional B-spline registration for chest CT images [12]. Eppenhof *et al* proposed a similar method using U-net. They showed the times per registration were 0.58 ± 0.07 s (deep learning-based) and 13.8 ± 5.7 min (B-spline-based) [13].

Finally, for (3) unsupervised transformation estimation, this method is not necessary to prepare ground truth data as described in methods (1) and (2). To our knowledge, the deep learning network for deformable image registration (DIRNet) proposed by Vos *et al* is the first deep learning method for end-to-end unsupervised DIR [14]. The DIRNet takes pairs of fixed and moving images as inputs, and it outputs moving images deformed to the fixed images (figure 4.10). The DIRNet consists of a convolutional neural network (ConvNet) regressor, a spatial transformer, and a resampler. The ConvNet analyzes a pair of fixed and moving images and outputs parameters for the spatial transformer, which generates the DVF. Since training of the DIRNet is unsupervised, this method is not trained with

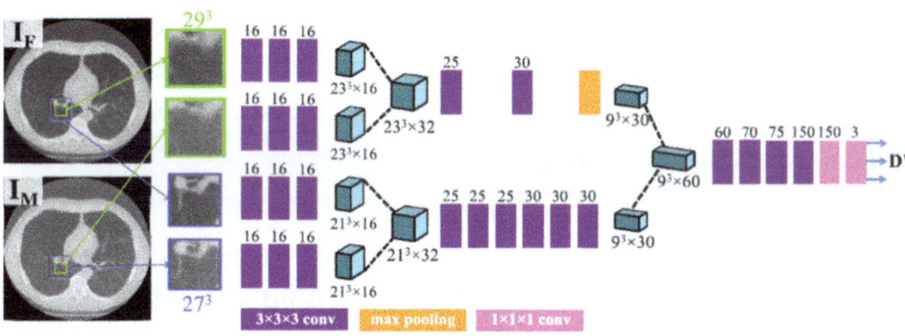

Figure 4.9. CNN architecture for supervised transformation estimation based on ResNet [12], copyright (2017) with permission of Springer.

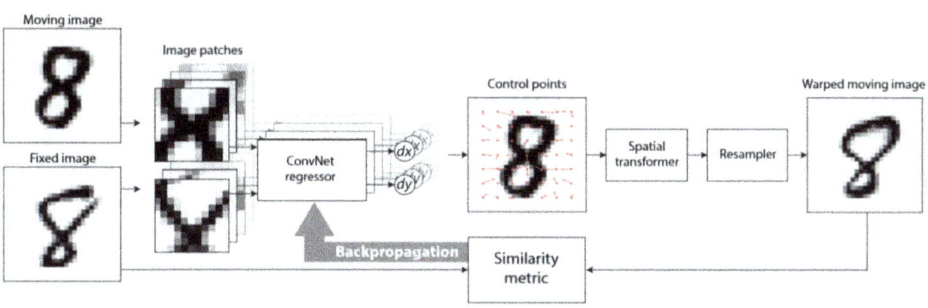

Figure 4.10. Basic framework for unsupervised transformation estimation using DIRNet [14], copyright (2017) with permission of Springer.

known DVFs, but learns to register images by directly optimizing the similarity metric between the fixed and the moving images. In addition, a trained DIRNet is able to perform DIR non-iteratively on unseen data. They showed that registration with DIRNet is as accurate as conventional DIR method with substantially shorter exclusion times for Cardiac cine MR scans.

4.4.2.2 Intrinsic limitations

Supervised learning-based methods, including the deep similarity metric and supervised transformation estimation, have great potential for improving the DIR accuracy and registration time. However, generally, it is hard to obtain the large amount of the ground truth of transformation. To tackle this issue, several studies created the synthetic ground truth data using various approaches. For example, Sokooti *et al* [12] generated synthetic DVFs with varying spatial frequency and amplitude, aiming to represent the range of displacements that can be seen in real images: (1) creating a vector field with the size of the input image and initializing it with zero vectors; (2) randomly selecting points in the DVF and randomly assigning three values to the displacement vector in the some ranges; (3) smoothing the DVF with a Gaussian kernel with a standard deviation of low, medium, and high values. It is important how close the synthetic ground truth data is to the real patient image. Thus, we need to understand that the residual error between the synthetic and real patient CT images may reduce the final DIR accuracy.

Regarding the unsupervised learning-based method, similarity metrics used as the loss function to perform the network leaning are still inefficient. Most unsupervised learning-based methods have been successful for the same modality images (e.g., CT-CT), but they didn't work well for different modality images (e.g., CT-MR).

4.4.3 Practical implementation of AI

4.4.3.1 Patient recognition, image acquisition range, auto-positioning

Patient recognition for medical image acquisition, automatic determination of image acquisition range, and auto-positioning have already been realized by the 3D camera integrated in the imaging device (e.g., CT scanner) and AI technology (e.g., Siemens SOMATOM X.cite, GE Revolution Maximana). This technology is common not only in radiotherapy but also in diagnostics. These systems use a 3D camera to detect the patient's body surface. Then they use this information and AI technology to determine the optimal image acquisition range and patient position for each patient. Saltybaeva *et al* evaluated the automatic individualized patient positioning using a 3D camera implemented in a CT scanner (SOMATOM Edge Plus; Siemens Healthineers, Forchheim, Germany) which allows for accurate patient centering by comparing with manual positioning [15]. The 3D depth sensor of the camera employs infrared light to measure the distance between objects and the camera. A virtual patient Avatar is fitted to the depth data and the geometric center of the Avatar is used to automatically set the vertical table position for the LR scan. Moreover, the workflow also allows the horizontal table position and the LR scan range based on body landmarks detected by the 3D camera image and the selected scan protocol to be set. They showed that automatic patient positioning based on the 3D camera reduced the average offset in vertical table position from 19 mm to 7 mm for chest and from 18 mm to 4 mm for abdomen CT. In addition, Booij *et al* also evaluated the accuracy of automatic patient positioning using Siemens's prototype system (figure 4.11). They showed that this system outperformed manual poisoning by radiographers [16].

As a different use of AI in the extension of patient recognition technology, it has been proposed to predict sudden movements during radiotherapy irradiation from the patient's facial expression. In recent years, surface guided radiation therapy (SGRT) using optical surface scanning for patient positioning, intra-fraction motion monitoring and respiratory gating techniques has been clinically used. In general, SGRT systems use a combination of a projector and one or several camera units to register a real-time 3D surface of the patients. This technology is a new technology that predicts the movement of the patient by using a camera, and has great potential for improving the clinical outcome of radiotherapy.

Specifically, the method proposed by Kim *et al* is to predict the next movement by the image of the patient's facial expression into deep learning [17]. They input 2D images of the facial expressions of 447 patients into the CNN with three convolutional layers to predict eight types of facial expression (natural, angry, contemptuous, disgusted, frightened, happy, sad, and surprised). The prediction accuracy was 85.6% in the test data of 10 patients, showing relatively good prediction accuracy (figure 4.12).

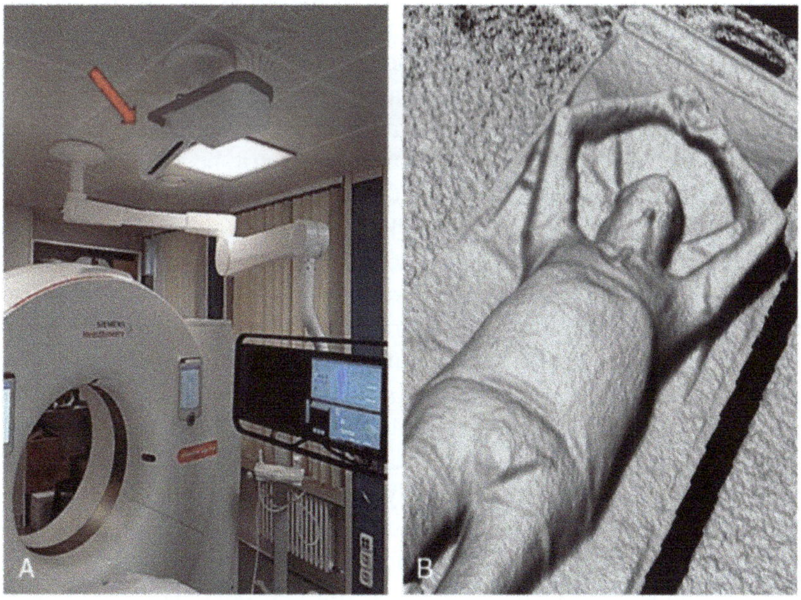

Figure 4.11. The 3D camera (red arrow) is placed above the CT table (a). 3D surface image of patient obtained with the 3D depth camera (b). Reprinted with permission from [15], copyright (2018) Wolters Kluwer Health Inc. All rights reserved.

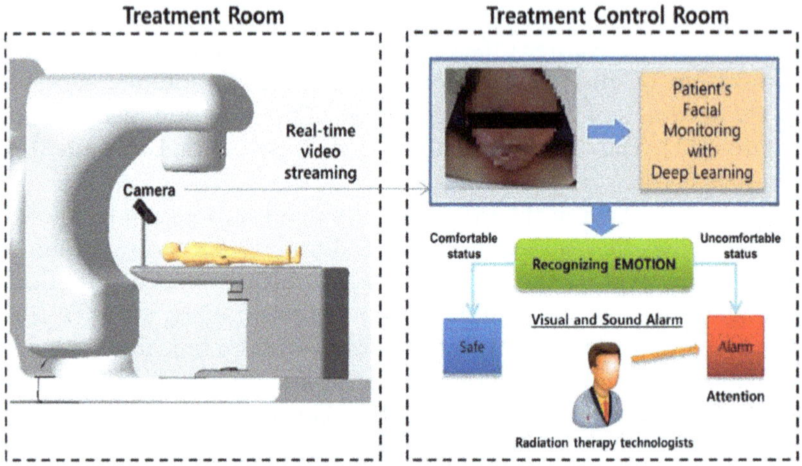

Figure 4.12. A facial expression monitoring system for patients in a radiation treatment room [17] John Wiley & Sons, copyright 2020 The Authors. Journal of Applied Clinical Medical Physics published by Wiley Periodicals, Inc. on behalf of American Association of Physicists in Medicine.

4.4.3.2 Optimal image acquisition setting regarding radiation exposure for CT

According to ALARA theory, radiation exposure should be as low as possible for the purpose of image acquisition in areas such as dose calculation, image registration, and diagnostic imaging. For dose calculation, auto-exposure control is generally applied to image acquisition for CT simulation purposes. However, the size of the patient should be taken into account and radiation exposure should be controlled due to patient size because of image quality, i.e., low signal-to-noise ratio. If the patient's body is large, the dose is increased, and if it is small, the dose is reduced. For image registration, when registration with bone is used, radiation exposure would be reduced because bone structure is visible even at low radiation doses. In contrast, when registration with soft tissue is used, radiation exposure would not be reduced because image quality the same as image acquisition for CT simulation is necessary.

In that situation, some neural networks (NN) have been proposed for image translation from low-dose CT images to normal-dose CT images [18]. Since NN can effectively grab many features from the pixel level through a hierarchical framework, image to image regression could be done for this purpose. The NN focusses on noise reduction, so-called denoising. CT images taken at low doses in advance and CT images taken at normal doses are prepared. In cases where preparing these CT images is difficult, another approach is available, that of simulated noise, e.g. Poisson noise, is added to a normal-dose sinogram and then CT image reconstruction is performed. Since it is difficult to increase training data easily, image patches are made to increase the training data as shown in figure 4.13. Because the role of the NN is denoising and the structure information of CT image is not necessary unlike organ segmentation, the splitted technique is efficient to increase training data. However, the predicted (denoised) image patch should be merged into the final image having original image size.

The network architecture consists of an auto-encoder with multiple convolution layers with skip connections regarding residual network. When the convolution

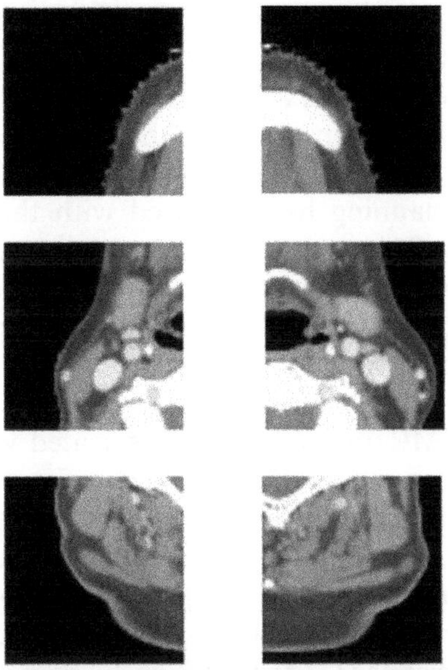

Figure 4.13. Image patches splitted from original CT image.

layer is applied to the input image several times, subtle image information such as image noise on the CT image will disappear and then the input image will be blurred. Therefore, the skip connection technique might be useful to maintain image features of the input image toward those of the output image. Owing to this network, low-dose CT images can be translated into normal-dose CT images, it will lead to reduced radiation exposure doses in patients. The proposed network is available online here (https://github.com/SSinyu/RED-CNN).

4.4.3.3 CT to MRI translation, MRI to CT translation, image deformation

CT to MR translation and MR to CT translation techniques are already clinically used. It should be noted that the method is an image deformation (DIR)-based method, not an AI-based method. The CT to MR translation technique can be used for electron density (ED) mapping by performing the DIR of CT image to MR image, resulting in MR-based dose calculation. This is used to create the MR-only treatment plan with a hybrid treatment device combining MRI with Linac (i.e., MR-Linac). The MR-Linac has recently been introduced and begun to be used clinically [19]. This system can obtain the MR image and create the MR-based treatment planning prior to treatment. The MR image allows for the accurate visualization of day-to-day changes in size, position, and deformation of tumors and organs at risk (OAR), enabling online adaptive radiotherapy (ART). Online ART where daily acquired images are used for re-optimization of the treatment plan prior to each fraction delivery is the optimal ART strategy to account for inter-fractional motion. Next, regarding the MR to CT translation technique, this technique can be used as an auxiliary image in CT-based delineation process by performing the DIR of the diagnostic or simulation MR image to the treatment planning CT image. As a result, it is possible to create accurate contours of the target and OARs with a combination of CT and MR images. Specifically, we can use the technique to delineate the clinical target volume (CTV) in the image-guided radiotherapy (e.g., prostate and head and neck).

In the first topics, CT to MRI translation, the utilization of AI has been actively studied. Recently, the amount of research on MR guided radiotherapy (MRgRT) based on the MR-only planning has increased with the development of clinical applications of MR-linac. The two MR-Linac system are commercially available: Unity (Elekta, Stockholm, Sweden) and MRIdian (ViewRay Inc., Oakwood, USA). Figure 4.14 shows an example of MR-based treatment planning with Monaco (Elekta, Stockholm, Sweden) for Unity.

The important thing is that MR image is not directly used for dose calculation since voxel intensities of MR image are not associated with the ED of tissues. In other words, CT images can create the CT-ED conversion table due to association between CT value and ED, but MR images cannot create this table.

Dose calculation cannot be performed unless ED is assigned to each voxel in the MR image in some way. At present, the following two methods have been proposed and clinically used: one is the method of assigning a representative ED (e.g., the average ED value of each organ in the planned CT image) to each organ, and the other is the method of mapping the ED by the DIR of the planning CT image to the MR image (this method was explained in the first topics) [20]. The drawback of the former method is that only simple ED mapping is possible, and accurate ED is not assigned to each voxel. The

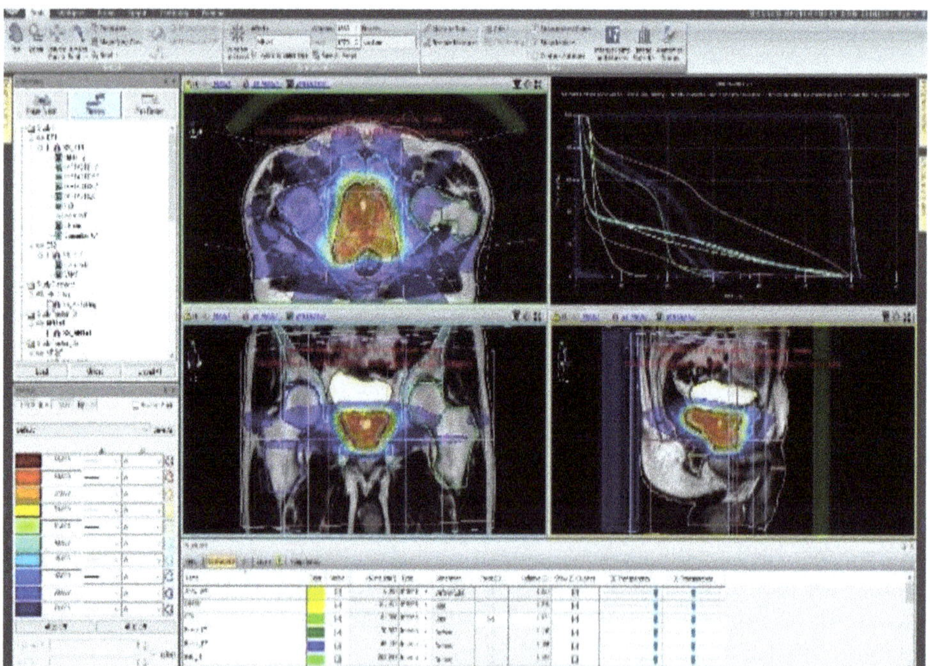

Figure 4.14. Example treatment planning with MR and dose distribution.

drawback of the latter method is that the DIR may not achieve sufficient registration accuracy due to multi-modality registration, resulting in poor ED mapping accuracy.

To improve the accuracy of MR-only dose calculation, deep learning-based synthetic CT generation has been proposed [21, 23]. Han *et al* proposed this method using U-net for the first time [23]. Figure 4.15 shows their proposed CNN model which is similar to U-net model. A lot of paired CT and MR images are prepared, and the CNN model was training using this dataset. The trained CNN model can generate the synthetic CT image from the input of MR image.

Chen *et al* also proposed the U-net-based CNN model for generating the synthetic CT image in pelvic region [21]. The example images are shown in figure 4.16. Images A, B, C and D are the input MR image, the actual CT image,

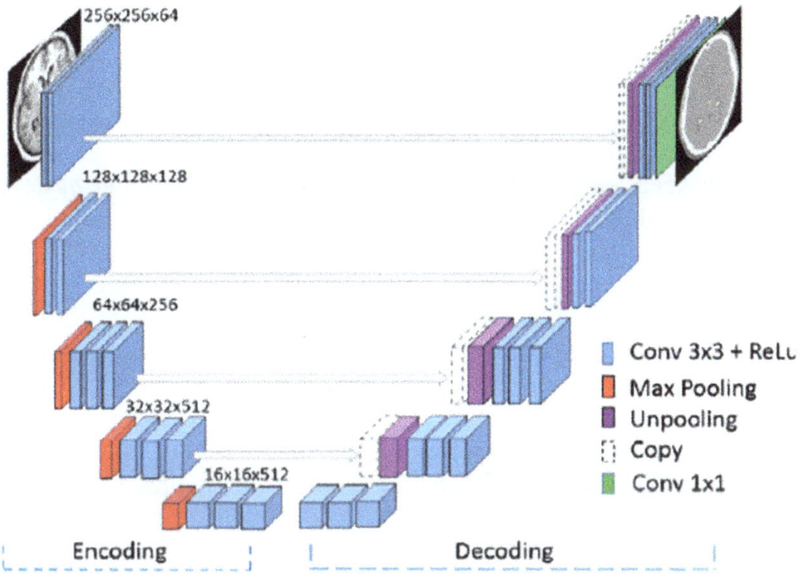

Figure 4.15. Overall architecture of the proposed deep learning-based synthetic CT generation method [23] John Wiley & Sons, copyright 2017 American Association of Physicists in Medicine.

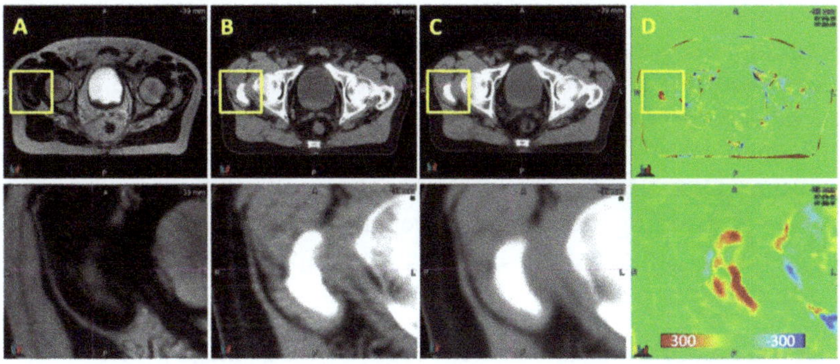

Figure 4.16. Representative synthetic image generated by deep learning [21] John Wiley & Sons, copyright 2017 American Association of Physicists in Medicine.

the synthetic CT, and the subtraction image between image B and C. The synthetic CT image generated by deep learning (image C) was considerably similar to the actual CT image (image B). They showed that mean absolute error were 29.96 ± 4.87 HU (U-net) and 38.9 ± 4.81 HU (DIR-based method), respectively, suggesting that U-net-based technique could improve the accuracy of MR-only planning. They also faced the issue that the ED map in bone region could not be estimated correctly due to insufficient training data sets. This may be due to the large variation in ED within the bone region among patients. Han *et al* mentioned the different issue that there was non-negligible registration error between CT and MR images in some cases [23]. This residual error may reduce the accuracy of synthetic CT image.

4.4.3.4 Image quality improvement

4.4.3.4.1 Noise reduction

Noise reduction (so-called image denozing) is an important topic in medical images including CT and MR images, and deep learning techniques have received much attention in the area of image denoising. Recently, various image denoising techniques with deep learning have been proposed [24]. Zhang *et al* developed a deep learning-based denoiser, the denoising convolutional neural networks (DnCNNs) that were trained with pairs of noisy- and noise-only images. Their denoiser improved the signal-to-noise ratio (SNR) of noisy images by removing noise components [25]. Chen *et al* combined the auto-encoder, deconvolution network, and shortcut connections into the residual encoder–decoder CNN (RED-CNN). They performed patch based training which helps to improve the results [26]. AI converts low-dose CT images to high-quality scans. Commercial systems equipped with these deep learning-based image denozing technique have already appeared. (e.g., AiCE (Advanced Intelligent Clear-IQ Engine, Cannon)).

4.4.3.4.2 Motion artifact reduction

CT and MR image images often have artifacts due to patient movement. Therefore, motion artifact reduction using AI has been proposed in various clinical sites, such as the brain and liver. Pawar *et al* developed the CNN-based motion correction in 3D MPRAGE image (MocoNet) for the brain. The network was an encoder–decoder CNN architecture where the encoder decomposed the motion corrupted images into a set of feature maps. The feature maps were then combined by the decoder network to generate a motion-corrected image [27]. In addition, Tamada *et al* also proposed a motion artifact reduction for DCE-MRI of the liver using DnCNN-based network with multi-channel input and output (figure 4.17). A training dataset was generated by simulating the respiratory motion. The results indicated the Deep learning approach possessed the ability to remove artifacts [28].

4.4.3.4.3 Reduction of contrast-enhanced region on CT image

CT simulation for treatment plan uses contrast enhance medium to enhance tumor regions more clearly in head and neck, esophagus, liver, and so on. First,

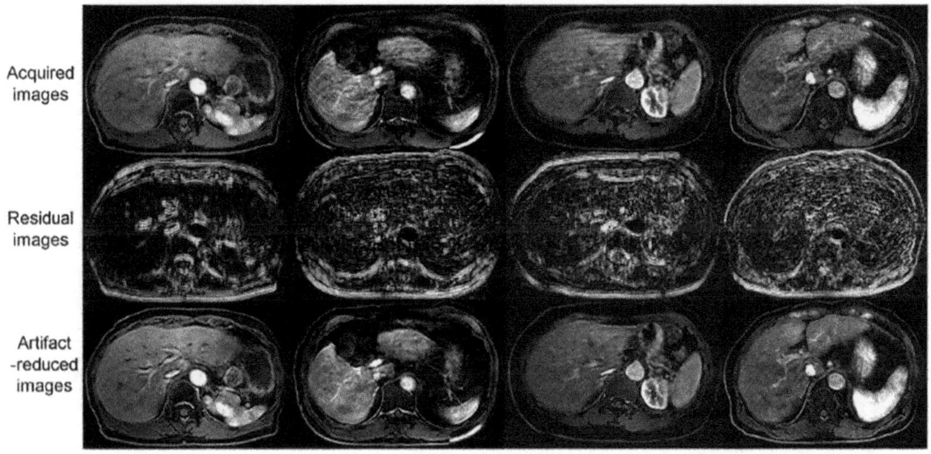

Figure 4.17. Examples of acquired and artifact-reduced images. motion artifacts in the images (upper row) were reduced (lower row) using the deep learning-based technique. The residual components are shown in the middle row. Republished from [28], with permission of MRMS.

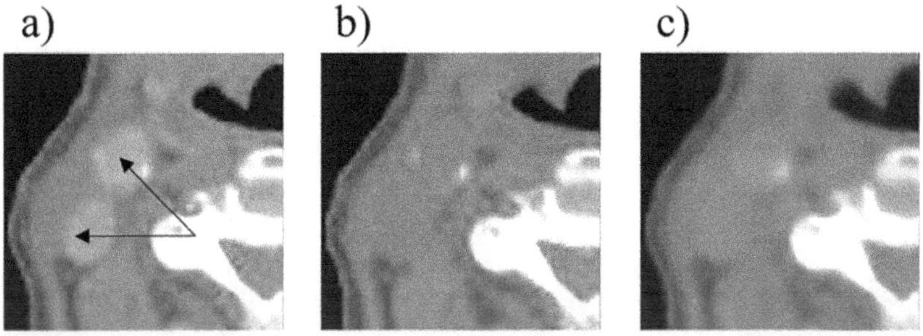

Figure 4.18. CT images of contrast-enhanced image (a), reference non-contrast-enhanced image (b), and predicted non-contrast-enhanced image (c).

non-contrast-enhanced CT images are taken, followed by contrast-enhanced CT images are taken as a secondary image. In terms of radiation exposure for the examination the patient is exposed twice to image acquisition. To reduce radiation exposure as much as possible, convolution neural network for this purpose, that is reduction of contrast-enhanced region, has been proposed [29]. According to the approach, the patient has only one CT examination with contrast-enhanced medium, which results in reduction of radiation exposure.

The proposed neural network is based on residual network, the so-called ResNet [30]. Figure 4.18(a) shows a non-contrast-enhanced image. Figure 4.18(c) was predicted by the proposal neural network. Contrast-enhanced regions indicated by black arrows have been reduced contrast enhance. The predicted non-contrast-enhanced CT image has also been used for dose calculation with comparable dose uncertainty when using reference non-contrast-enhanced CT image.

4.4.3.5 Challenges and future work

4.4.3.5.1 Time reduction of CBCT image acquisition

In CT simulation, high-speed helical scanning is possible, so imaging is possible in a short time. In contrast CBCT image acquisition used for image registration takes 30 s to 1 min, the gantry rotates 200° or 360° for imaging. It is more comfortable for the patient to take a picture in as short a time as possible, so that the patient motion during imaging is also reduced. In future radiation therapy, it is expected that the patient will be placed on a treatment couch from CT imaging, treatment planning, and irradiation. In that case, it is necessary to aim to shorten the time at each step of CT imaging, time to delineation of organs on CT images, and time to formulate treatment plans. T0 shorten the time of CBCT imaging, we will introduce a study that aims at image reconstruction equivalent to full scanning using neural network by reconstructing images at a limited rotation angle.

Figure 4.19(a) is a CT image of a treatment plan. The projection image was created from the planning CT images. In this case, 45 projection images were created by gantry rotation of 1° each. A CBCT image was reconstructed by Feldkamp–Davis–Kress algorithm [31] using the 45 projection images, which is shown in figure 4.19(c). Figure 4.19(c) was used as input data, and figure 4.19(a) was used as output data. So that the convolution neural network using U-net predicted CT image as if an image acquisition was performed by a full gantry rotation shown in figure 4.19(d). Typically, it takes one minute to acquire projection images of full gantry rotation, whereas it takes as little as 7.5 s to acquire projection images. This can save significant time.

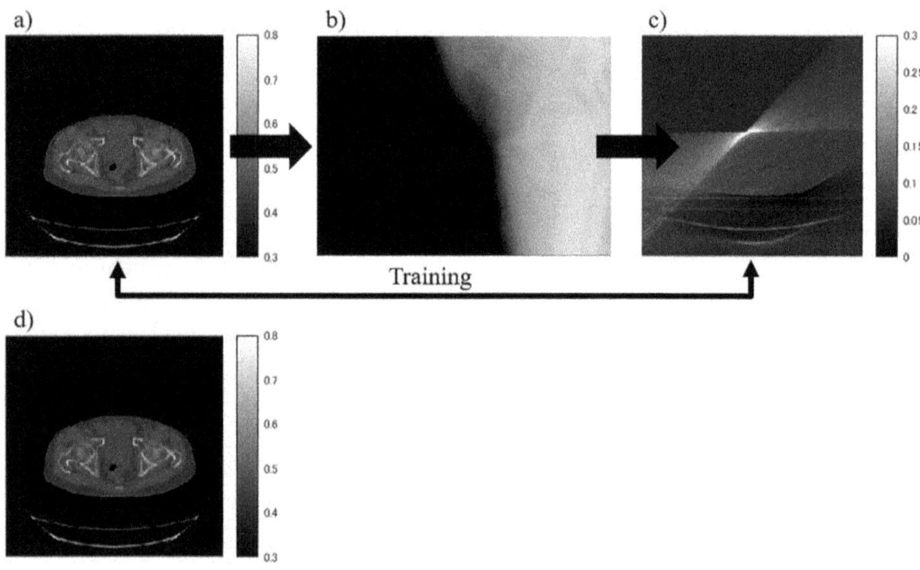

Figure 4.19. Images of reference CT image (a), projection image (b), CBCT image under a limited rotation angle (c), and predicted CT image (d).

4.4.3.5.2 Challenges for AI-based DIR

Regarding the image deformation, first, supervised transformation estimation showed the great potential for improving the DIR accuracy. However, generally, it is hard to obtain the large amount of the ground truth of transformation. To tackle this issue, several studies created the synthetic ground truth data using various approaches [32–34]. Sokooti *et al* generated the synthetic DVFs for thoracic CT images using varying spatial frequency and amplitude, aiming to represent the range of displacements that can be seen in real images: (1) creating a vector field with the size of the input image and initializing it with zero vectors; (2) randomly selecting P points in the DVF and randomly assigning three values to the displacement vector in the range $[-\theta, +\theta]$; (3) smoothing the DVF with a Gaussian kernel with a standard deviation of σ. Low, medium and high frequency deformations are generated using the settings $\sigma = 35$, $P = 80$, $\theta = 8$; $\sigma = 25$, $P = 100$, $\theta = 8$; and $\sigma = 20$, $P = 100$, $\theta = 8$ [32]. These approaches have the great potential for improving the DIR accuracy of supervised learning-based registration, but the concern with these approaches is how close the generated virtual CT is to a real patient's CT. For organs that have a large deformation in the local region, such as the rectum and small bowel, it may be difficult to mechanically generate the synthetic DVF. In the future, it will be necessary to develop a useful method of augmentation for DVF.

In addition, regarding the unsupervised transformation estimation, previous studies mainly used the similarity metric as the loss estimation in learning process [35, 36]. This method faces the same issue as the conventional intensity-based DIR. That is, generally, it is difficult to define the accurate similarity of the moving and fixed images in multi-modality registration. Mutual information is commonly used as the similarity metric in multi-modality registration, but intensity-based MR-CT DIR often does not work well. In the future work, it will be necessary to develop a different method for unsupervised learning-based registration.

References

[1] Hong T S, Tomé W A and Chappell R J *et al* 2005 The impact of daily setup variations on head-and-neck intensity-modulated radiation therapy *Int. J. Radiat. Oncol. Biol. Phys.* **61** 779–88

[2] White P, Yee C K and Shan L C *et al* 2014 A comparison of two systems of patient immobilization for prostate radiotherapy *Radiat. Oncol.* **9** 29

[3] Ueda Y, Teshima T and Cárdenes H *et al* 2017 Evaluation of initial setup errors of two immobilization devices for lung stereotactic body radiation therapy (SBRT) *J. Appl. Clin. Med. Phys.* **18** 62–8

[4] Pisani L, Lockman D and Jaffray D *et al* 2000 Setup error in radiotherapy: on-line correction using electronic kilovoltage and megavoltage radiographs *Int. J. Radiat. Oncol. Biol. Phys.* **47** 825–39

[5] Goldsowrthy S and McGrail S 2014 Prone belly board device training improves geometric setup accuracy in lower GI radiotherapy *J. Radiother. Pract.* **13** 302–9

[6] Söderberg M and Gunnarsson M 2010 Automatic exposure control in computed tomography—an evaluation of systems from different manufactures *Acta Radiol.* **51** 625–34

[7] NCRP 1990 Implementation of the principle of as low as reasonably achievable (ALARA) for medical and dental personnel. NCRP Report 107

[8] Oh S and Kim S 2017 Deformable image registration in radiation therapy *Radiat oncol.* **35** 101

[9] Brock K K, Mutic S and McNutt T R *et al* 2017 Use of image registration and fusion algorithms and techniques in radiotherapy: report of the AAPM radiation therapy committee task group no. 132 *Med. Phys.* **44** e43–6

[10] Weistrand O and Svensson S 2015 The ANACONDA algorithm for deformable image registration in radiotherapy *Med. Phys.* **42** 40–53

[11] Cheng X, Zhang L and Zheng Y 2018 Deep similarity learning for multimodal medical images *Comput. Methods Biomech. Biomed. Eng. Imagi. Visualizat.* **6** 248–52

[12] Sokooti H, de Vos B and Berendsen F *et al* 2017 *Nonrigid Image Registration Using Multi-scale 3D Convolutional Neural Networks* (Cham: Springer Int. Publishing) pp 232–9

[13] Eppenhof K A J and Pluim J P W 2019 Pulmonary CT registration through supervised learning with convolutional neural networks *IEEE Trans. Med. Imaging* **38** 1097–105

[14] de Vos B D, Berendsen F F and Viergever M A *et al* 2017 End-to-end unsupervised deformable image registration with a convolutional neural network *arXiv:1704.06065*

[15] Saltybaeva N, Schmidt B and Wimmer A *et al* 2018 Precise and automatic patient positioning in computed tomography: avatar modeling of the patient surface using a 3-dimensional camera *Invest Radiol.* **53** 641–6

[16] Booij R, Budde R P J and Dijkshoorn M L *et al* 2019 Accuracy of automated patient positioning in CT using a 3D camera for body contour detection *Eur Radiol.* **29** 2079–88

[17] Kim K H, Park K and Kim H *et al* 2020 Facial expression monitoring system for predicting patient's sudden movement during radiotherapy using deep learning *J. Appl. Clin. Med. Phys.* **21** 191–9

[18] Chen H, Zhang Y and Kaira M K *et al* 2017 Low-dose CT with a residual encorder–decorder convolutional neural network *IEEE Trans. Med. Imag.* **36** 2524–35

[19] Raaymakers B W, Jurgenliemk-Schulz I M and Bol G H *et al* 2017 First patients treated with a 1.5 T MRI-Linac: clinical proof of concept of a high-precision, high-field MRI guided radiotherapy treatment *Phys. Med. Biol.* **62** L41–50

[20] Hunt A, Hanson I and Dunlop A *et al* 2020 Feasibility of magnetic resonance guided radiotherapy for the treatment of bladder cancer *Clin. Transl. Radiat. Oncol.* **25** 46–51

[21] Chen S, Qin A and Zhou D *et al* 2018 Technical note: U-net generated synthetic CT images for magnetic resonance imaging-only prostate intensity-modulated radiation therapy treatment planning *Med. Phys.* **45** 5659–65

[22] Arabi H, Dowling J A and Burgos N *et al* 2018 Comparative study of algorithms for synthetic CT generation from MRI: consequences for MRI-guided radiation planning in the pelvic region *Med. Phys.* **45** 5218–33

[23] Han X 2017 MR-based synthetic CT generation using a deep convolutional neural network method *Med. Phys.* **44** 1408–19

[24] Shan H, Padole A and Homayounieh F *et al* 2019 Competitive performance of a modularized deep neural network compared to commercial algorithms for low-dose CT image reconstruction *Nat. Mach. Intell.* **1** 269–76

[25] Zhang K, Zuo W and Chen Y *et al* 2017 Beyond a gaussian denoiser: residual learning of deep CNN for image denoising *IEEE Trans. Image Process.* **26** 3142–55

[26] Chen H, Zhang Y and Kalra M K *et al* 2017 Low-dose CT with a residual encoder–decoder convolutional neural network *IEEE Trans. Med. Imaging* **36** 2524–35

[27] Pawar K, Chen Z and Shah N J *et al* 2018 MoCoNet: Motion correction in 3D MPRAGE images using a convolutional neural network approach arXiv:1807.10831

[28] Tamada D, Kromrey M L and Ichikawa S *et al* 2020 Motion artifact reduction using a convolutional neural network for dynamic contrast enhanced MR imaging of the liver *Magn. Reson. Med. Sci.* **19** 64–76

[29] Sumida I, Magome T and Kitamori H *et al* 2019 Deep convolutional neural network for reduction of contrast-enhanced region on CT images *J. Radiat. Res.* **60** 586–94

[30] He K, Zhang X and Ren S *et al* Deep residual learning for image recognition arXiv:1512.03385

[31] Feldkamp L A, Davis L C and Kress J W 1984 Practical cone-beam algorithm *J. Opt. Soc. Am.* A **1** 612–9

[32] Sokooti H, de Vos B and Berendsen F *et al* 2017 *Nonrigid Image Registration Using Multi-scale 3D Convolutional Neural Networks* (Cham: Springer Int. Publishing) pp 232–9

[33] Eppenhof K A J and Pluim J P W 2019 Pulmonary CT registration through supervised learning with convolutional neural networks *IEEE Trans. Med. Imaging* **38** 1097–105

[34] Ito M and Ino F 2018 An automated method for generating training sets for deep learning based image registration **2** 140–7

[35] Dalca A V, Balakrishnan G and Guttag J *et al* 2018 Unsupervised learning for fast probabilistic diffeomorphic registration arXiv:1805.04605

[36] Cao X, Yang J and Wang L *et al* 2018 Deep learning based inter-modality image registration supervised by intra-modality similarity arXiv:1804.10735

IOP Publishing

Artificial Intelligence in Radiation Therapy

Iori Sumida

Chapter 5

Organ delineation

Xiao Ying and Men Kuo

5.1 Introduction to organ delineation in radiotherapy

5.1.1 Organ delineation in the radiation therapy process

5.1.1.1 Variations in the delineation

5.1.1.1.1 Standardization of the definitions

Radiotherapy has advanced substantially since the discovery and application of radiation for medical treatment. Radiation treatment planning and administration has advanced rapidly from two-dimensional planning and administration to volumetric three-dimensional conformal radiation treatment, intensity-modulated radiation therapy (IMRT), and proton beam radiation treatment (PBT). The technologies have permitted dose optimization to target quantities while avoiding harm to the organ at risk. Modern radiation is predicated on the identification of targets and essential structures. Under-contouring the target may reduce the efficiency of radiation, resulting in recurrence and reduced survival. Under-contouring the OAR results in less OAR sparing, which may result in increased or unanticipated toxicity; over-contouring the OAR leads to unnecessary dose decreases to the target. Contouring mistakes may result in unintended dose distribution to an OAR, resulting in unanticipated toxicity throughout the patient's treatment procedure.

The quantitative analyses of normal tissue effects in the clinic (QUANTEC) review proposed OAR tolerances and defined OAR constraints [1], in conjunction with the hypofractionated radiation therapy/SBRT (HyTEC) updates [2], demonstrates the critical impact of treatment decisions impact upon patient outcomes.

The accuracy of the definitions of treatment objects impacts clinical research in radiation therapy and therefore its understanding and advancement. Through analysis of high-level evidence generated from well-conducted prospective clinical trials, or retrospective evaluation of real-world data extracted from big data repositories, the dosimetric, toxicity, and endpoint reporting parameters from these datasets inform the development of normal tissue complication probability (NTCP) models and tumor control probability models (TCP) and define dosimetric constraints for future radiation therapy planning. Variability in the reporting standards, inconsistencies in nomenclature and inconsistency in contouring guidance may increase contour variability. Consistency and accuracy in structure nomenclature and contouring guidance not only minimizes variation but also improves workflow and safety, including facilitation of the generation of robust auto-segmentation models [3].

Extensive organizational efforts have been undertaken for the standardization of the structure definitions. Examples include Standardizing Nomenclatures in Radiation Oncology, the report of AAPM Task Group 263, which provided standard structure names across image processing and treatment planning system platforms; nomenclature for dosimetric data (e.g., dose/volume histogram [DVH]-based metrics); templates of an initial subset; formalism for nomenclature schema which can accommodate the addition of other structures [4]. The Global Harmonization Group presented organ at risk delineation guidelines for radiation therapy clinical trials for 73 OARs with nomenclature and peer-reviewed descriptions [3]. Examples of standardization for specific organs include the establishment of the Danish Comprehensive Cancer Center Onco-Cardiology society to optimize Danish research in cardiac toxicity after cancer treatment, to develop and validate national delineation guidelines for the heart and cardiac substructures [5].

5.1.1.1.2 Inter- and intra-observer variation

The variations in definition of structures could be subjective or objective. There have been extensive reports on the differences between the contours by the same clinician in a span of time and between multiple clinicians over the same structure.

Peer review is incorporated in the radiotherapy process for the quality and safety of patient treatments. The process is defined as the evaluation of scientific, academic, or professional work by others working in the same field. The reported change of target volume and critical structure definition can occur in over 30% of the cases. The variations are largely dependent on the treatment technique, disease site, and physician experience [6].

In the Danish report quoted above, the agreement level of heart and cardiac substructures were reported in the Dice coefficient. The Dice similarity coefficient (DSC), also known as the Sørensen–Dice index or simply Dice coefficient, is a statistical tool which measures the similarity between two sets of data. The Dice coefficient is 2 * the area of overlap divided by the total number of pixels in both images. The detailed definition is included in the following sections. DSC was 0.78–0.96 for the heart and the four cardiac chambers. For the four substructures of the left ventricle, the median DSC was 0.35–0.57. The coronary arteries were contoured in ten segments, with the best agreement for the left anterior descending coronary artery segments, with a median distance between the arteries ranging from 2.4–4.4 mm. The median variation was 3.7–12.8 mm for the right coronary artery segments and 3.7–6.2 mm for the left circumflex coronary artery segments, with the most pronounced inter-observer variation in the distal segment for all three coronary arteries [5].

The extent of inter-observer variability in the delineation of head and neck cancer (HNC) was reported for the clinical target volume of the primary tumour (CTVp) and elective nodal neck (CTVe). The volume, Dice similarity coefficient (DSC) and median Hausdorff distance (HD, defined in later sections) were measured and calculated. The median DSC for CTVe ranged between 0.67 and 0.88 and HD50 between 1.7 mm and 2.8 mm. The median DSC and HD50 for CTVp ranged between 0.51 and 0.79, and 2.8 mm and 4.1 mm respectively [7]. Extensive inter-observer variations were reported on organ at risk, with those for parotid glands (DSC 0.77–0.91, HD 5.0–10.7 mm), brainstem (DSC 0.66–0.92), eyeballs (DSC 0.83–0.95), optic chiasm/optic nerves (DSC 0.38–0.79), cochlea (DSC 0.37–0.78), and brachial plexus (DSC 0.26) [8].

Contouring pelvic anatomy for prostate cancer treatment can be highly variable among observers, with significant uncertainty in target delineation. Clinical target volume (CT and MR), bladder, and rectum contours showed excellent inter-observer agreement (DSC = 0.83 ± 0.05; 0.88 ± 0.05; 0.93 ± 0.03; 0.81 ± 0.07; 0.80 ± 0.06, respectively). Seminal vesicle contours were more variable (DSC = 0.73 ± 0.14), while colon and bowel bag contoured volumes displayed poor overlap (DSC = 0.58 ± 0.22; 0.67 ± 0.21) [9, 10].

5.1.1.1.3 Intrinsic limitations

To reach perfect agreement from inter- and intra-observers is difficult due to the intrinsic limitations of the data as input to the delineation process.

These limitations include image contrast between the structure and surrounding tissue, low spatial representations, and inconsistency in utilization of contrast agents.

Variability in size and shape between patients; variable appearance as a result of physiological changes (e.g. bladder filling or gas); motion effect; presence of treatment aid objects, such as fiducials in gold seeds or radiofrequency beacons can affect the image quality thereby the delineation consistency and quality of the structures [5, 10, 11].

5.1.2 Impact of delineation accuracies

5.1.2.1 Dosimetric effect

The significant inter- and intra-practitioner variability may exceed planning and setup errors and result in significant dosimetric impact for the patient. As an example, to illustrate the inter-clinician OAR delineation variability and its dosimetric impact, an international study included 32 different centres and delineated OARs on a single CT dataset. Significant variations in dose were found for parotid glands, brainstem, and spinal cord. This translated into differences in Dmean of parotids of up to 50% and to more than 20% in brainstem Dmax. With regard to PTV coverage, the plans were evaluated for V95—volume receiving 95% of prescribed dose; and D99—near minimum dose in PTV. The volumes differ by a mean of 8.7%, leading to a reduction in V95 of 7.2% ± 5.4% (1SD), and a mean reduction in D99 of 14.2 Gy. Even for DSC > 0.8 and mean contour distances

<1 mm, reductions in D99 of up to 11 Gy were observed. Similar variations are reported from other studies [12, 13].

5.1.2.2 Impact on treatment outcome
The quality of structure delineation is associated with radiotherapy outcome, affecting survival, local control, and toxicities from the treatments.

A meta study of clinical trials with reporting on radiotherapy quality linked accuracy of target and organ at risk segmentation with outcome with significant hazardous ratios for most of the studies chosen [14]. The survival impact could reach up to 20% from the lack of compliance with the protocol defined guidelines [15].

With more advanced radiotherapy technology, more precise radiotherapy ensures only delineated volumes are treated, as compared with conformational RT in which larger volumes received the prescription dose. Inferior delineation of the target not following guidelines risk recurrence from the treatment. This is demonstrated in a study that showed that not following the delineation recommendations seems to significantly increase the recurrence risk [16]. In the study, almost half of patients had non-compliant delineation, not following the delineation's recommendations.

5.2 Organ delineation methodologies

5.2.1 Automated image segmentation techniques and deep learning applications

Due to the critical nature of an accurate and efficient delineation process, significant research and development efforts have been made in the approaches, most notably approaches that automate the process and enhance over consistency. A selection of various automated strategies is discussed, as well as quantitative measurements for evaluating the delineation quality.

5.2.1.1 Methodologies

5.2.1.1.1 Classic auto-segmentation
The traditional automatic segmentation methods are derived from statistical evaluation/models of the image intensity, spatial textures and geometric shapes, or atlas-based models [17, 18]. Thresholding, region-based segmentation, edge detection, atlas-based segmentation, and model-based segmentation are among the topics covered in the following sections.

(1) Thresholding

Thresholding is a fundamental image segmentation technique that involves calculating one or more grayscale thresholds based on an image's grayscale properties [19]. To achieve image segmentation, the pixels in the image are grouped based on specified grayscale intervals. Global, local (adaptive), and optimal thresholding are types of variations. The goal of optimal thresholding is to find the best grayscale thresholds based on specific criterion functions. Thresholding is a very efficient method that takes very little computing. It is especially useful for images with contrasting gray levels between the target and the background, such as outlining lungs during radiation. Thresholding is also employed in image pre-processing. However, this method solely considers the grayscale qualities of pixels, leaving out spatial features and other relevant data. As a result, it is ineffective for identifying complex organs.

(2) Region-based segmentation

The process of zoning an image using similarity criteria is known as region-based segmentation [20]. Region splitting and growing, as well as water-shedding, are examples of variations. A set of seed points (individual pixels or small regions) is established first in region growth. The pixels or regions around the seed points that match particular growing requirements are then blended with the original seed points to create new seed points. This cycle is performed until a pre-set condition is met. Selecting seed places, establishing growing criteria, and establishing termination criteria are three essential components of region development. Grayscale, contour, color, and gradient information can all be used to determine the growth criterion. The ease of region growth makes it ideal for segmenting consistently connected targets. The downsides include its high noise sensitivity and the requirement for manual seed point confirmation.

A continuous image is separated into several sections using pre-set splitting and margin criteria in region splitting and merging. The target is then defined by combining the foreground regions. A quadtree decomposition divides regions with inconsistent properties into four equal subregions, which is the most prevalent form. Then, until no more subregions meet the splitting and merging requirements, surrounding subregions with similar features are constantly combined. Finally, to achieve segmentation, adjacent zones with similar properties are blended. The method of area splitting and merging is more complicated than the others. It is suitable for defining complex targets or scenarios where you don't have a lot of information.

The watershed segmentation approach uses topological ideas to segment an image into watersheds. Each local minimum value and the impacted region is represented by a catchment basin, and the grayscale value of each pixel in the image is represented by an altitude value. The margins of contiguous catchment basins constitute watersheds. As a result, the watersheds in an input image reflect the spots with the highest value. Watershed segmentation is a useful technique for finding continuous edges and distinguishing targets with fuzzily defined bounds. Excessive segmentation can, however, be caused by noise and small variations in grayscale value.

(3) Edge detection

Generally, changes in the grayscale values of pixels around the borders of distinct sections are more pronounced. Edge detection uses edge features to segment images and calculates gray levels and structural discontinuities [21]. Calculating derivatives can be used to detect discontinuities. The Roberts Cross, Prewitt, Sobel, Kirsch, and Robinson operators are common first-order differential operators, whereas the Marr–Hildreth, Canny, Laplacian, LOG, and DOG operators are common second-order differential operators. Edge detection is quick and precise. Broken edges in detail-intensive continuous and closed regions, on the other hand, are unavoidable. To accomplish segmentation operations, edge detection must be combined with postprocesses or other applicable algorithms.

(4) Atlas-based segmentation

Atlas-based contouring algorithms use a library of expert contoured images, with different organ sizes and shapes that represent the range of anatomic variations. Atlas-based auto-contouring uses image registration between an atlas image and the new image to calculate the transformation, which is used to transfer atlas contours onto the new image. Atlas-based methods vary in size and quality of atlas library, image-registration techniques (e.g., rigid or elastic), contour post-processing techniques (e.g., smoothing), and the number of atlases used for auto-contouring (e.g., single or multiple) [11, 17].

Atlas-based methods have become available in commercial radiation therapy software [11]. Two commercial systems that perform user-defined ABAS—Mirada's Workflow Box (WFB, Mirada Medical, Ltd., Oxford, UK) and MIM Maestro (MIM Software Inc., Cleveland, OH)—were used to automatically segment target structures [22]. Other commercial solutions are listed in table 5.1.

(5) Shape model-based segmentation

Shape characteristics and constraints are used in the shape model-based segmentation methodology to retrieve predetermined shapes or structures within images [23]. Active shape models, active appearance models, active contours, deformable templates, and level sets are common models used in this technique.

Table 5.1 contains a summary of commercially available methodologies. The traditional approaches have various drawbacks, the most significant of which is that they are incapable of dealing with big variations across images, such as those caused by organ motions or deformations. These strategies limit the final segmentation outcomes to anatomically plausible but less flexible shape or positions indicated by the models, resulting in segmentations that fail to meet clinical accuracy requirements [17].

5.2.1.1.2 AI powered delineation

The most recent approach to automated delineation involves artificial intelligence (AI). AI refers to the intelligence achieved by computer systems. machine learning (ML), a subcategory of AI, has been studied for decades because of the computer

Table 5.1. Common commercial automatic delineation software.

Developer	Name	Auto-delineation method
Varian	Eclipse (Smart Segmentation)	Atlas-based
MIM Software	MIM Maestro 6+	Atlas-based
Velocity	VelocityAI 3.0.1	Atlas-based
BrainLab	iPlan	Atlas-based
Dosisoft	IMAgo	Atlas-based
Mirada	RTx 1.4, Workflow box	Atlas-based
OSL	OnQ RTS	Atlas-based
Elekta	ABAS 2.01	Atlas- and shape model-based
Philips	SPICE 9.8	Atlas- and shape model-based
RaySearch	RayStation 4.0	Atlas- and shape model-based

system's capability of solving practical problems by learning from data. Deep learning (DL), a subcategory of ML, has achieved remarkable performance surpassing traditional ML approaches in recent years as a consequence of the availability of large-scale datasets, innovative DL technologies, advanced model training algorithms, as well as rapidly growing computing powers [24].

ML is a subcategory of methods within the broad scope of AI, with DL as a group of methods within ML.

The most commonly employed models in DL are deep neural networks (DNNs), which are a type of artificial neural network (ANN) [25] but with a large number of layers.

To date, a large number of DNN architectures have been designed for different applications. For example, convolutional neural networks (CNNs) proposed by LeCun *et al* [26] effectively use convolutional layers for image-related tasks. The convolutional computation utilizes a kernel and convolves with the previous layer's image data to produces new images, called feature images, and feeds them to the next layer. An activation function in a neural network defines how the weighted sum of the input is transformed into an output from a node or nodes in a layer of the network. Pooling layers provide an approach to down sampling feature maps by summarizing the presence of features in patches of the feature map. Two common pooling methods are average pooling and max pooling that summarize the average presence of a feature and the most activated presence of a feature respectively. This allows for the model to reduce computational cost and to view and analyse the images at multiple resolution scales. In addition to these layers, CNNs can still incorporate other operations such as fully-connected layers, batch/layer/instance/group normalizations, non-linear activations, etc. A fully-connected layer looks at what high-level features most strongly correlate to a particular class and has particular weights so that when we compute the products between the weights and the previous layer, we obtain the correct probabilities for the different classes.

Several variants of CNN model structures for classification have been proposed, such as AlexNet [27], VGGNet [28], and GoogleNet [29]. CNNs have also been employed widely for image-to-image translation tasks.

One of the most common applications of such CNNs is image segmentation, with segmented region maps as the output. The U-net [30] and its 3D variant, the V-net [31], are two prominent architectures for this task. The V-net was the first to add the Dice loss layer, which is now frequently used. Figure 5.1 shows the basic construction of U-net type architecture, which comprises a contracting path and an expansive path in the shape of the letter U. The contracting path decreases spatial while boosting feature information by convolution, activation, and pooling, whereas the expansive path executes up-convolutions of feature and spatial information with lateral concatenations of low and high-level feature maps. The architecture was released as open-source (https://lmb.informatik.uni-freiburg.de/resources/opensource/unet/) [8]. U-Net/V-net adopted the encoder–decoder network to accomplish neuronal structures segmentation and cell tracking tasks. An encoder–decoder neural network is a modular neural network that consists of an encoder network and a decoder network. Because of the multiple layers of convolutions and pooling

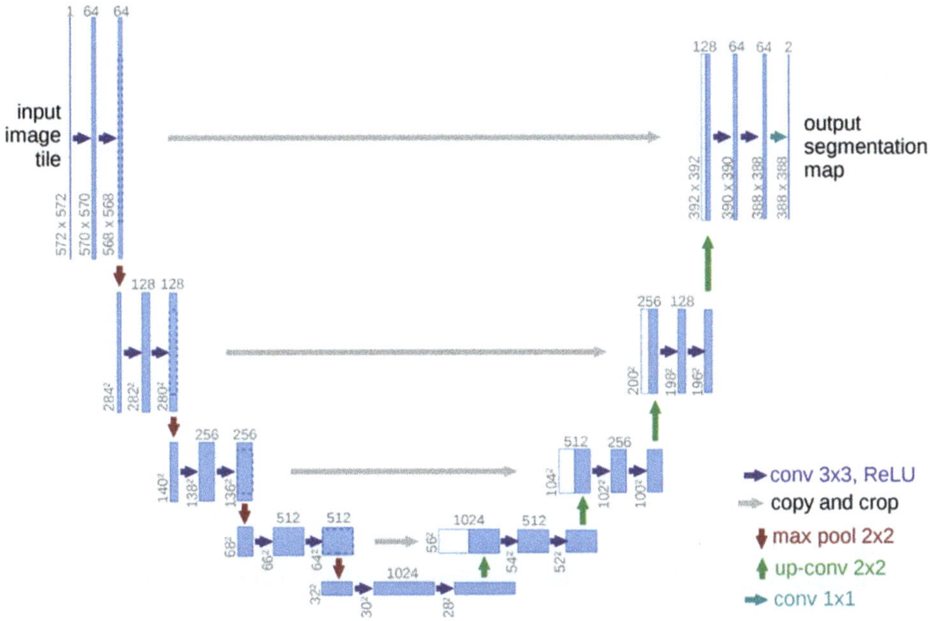

Figure 5.1. U-Net: convolutional networks for biomedical image segmentation. Reprinted from [71], copyright 2015, Springer International Publishing Switzerland. With permission of Springer.

operations to change image resolutions among layers, U-net's and V-net's architectures allow effective calculation and combination of both local and global features.

Many variations of these two networks have appeared in the literature, typically with modifications designed for the specific tasks of the studies [24, 32]. For example, DeepMedic11 employed a dual-path 3D CNN-based on dense patch ideas to deal with the high computational burden when training 3D CNN for brain lesion segmentation. DeepMedic13's two parallel convolutional paths allow for processing the input at multiple scales to achieve a large receptive field for classification while using small convolutional kernels that are associated with relatively low computational costs. It was released as open-source (https://biomedia.doc.ic.ac.uk/software/deepmed ic/), and extended to an augmented version for specific tasks, e.g., DeepVoxNet15 for head and neck disease site segmentation [8]. UNet++ connected the encoder and decoder networks by a series of dense skip connections to avoid eliminating the gap between encoder and decoder networks and obtained better performance than U-Net and wide U-Net on four segmentation datasets [33]. AnatomyNet was achieved by combining squeeze-and-excitation residual blocks into U-Net for segmenting OARs from head and neck CT images [11]. In order to improve the feature extraction, a 3D dual-path U-Net was used to segment the cancer region as well as critical structures [17, 27] DeepLabv3+, ResUNet, and DDCNN, (3D) fully convolutional DenseNet (FCDN) [33] have the standard encoder–decoder architecture. DeepLabv3+ has a shortcut connection that transfers low-level features from the encoder to the decoder. The model employs ResNet-50 as the encoder, using an atrous spatial pyramid pooling (ASPP) module aiming for high-level feature extraction and a concat-aggregation operator to integrate multiple-level features. ResUNet is inspired by the conventional UNet with modification to the encoder component that encodes target features at different abstraction levels and those features are passed to the decoder module via shortcut connections. Each level of features in the encoder and decoder were concatenated. Low-level features were used to generate the segmentation results. DDCNN has no shortcut connections between the encoder and decoder, which means that low-level information is not emphasized. In DDCNN, the sum aggregation operator is used to fuse the multiple scale features, which may lose information [18, 22, 34–38].

Other methodologies have been explored, sometimes combined with CNN, for the segmentation.

ReSeg [39], a structured prediction architecture, exploits the local generic features extracted by CNN and the capacity of recurrent neural networks (RNN) to retrieve distant dependencies to perform the task of semantic segmentation.

The mask R-CNN is an instance segmentation network [40]. This method identifies targets in images (frame location) before delineating the target (pixel classification). As a result, this method can be classified as a mixture of target identification and semantic segmentation. For target detection, faster R-CNNs are preferable, while FCNs are favoured for semantic segmentation. Mask R-CNN is an expansion of Faster R-CNN that uses the RoIAlign function for feature extraction instead of the RoIPooling function. The issue of misalignment caused by direct pooling is now resolved. Furthermore, this method uses a branch mask layer to identify boxes, followed by an FCN to classify the pixels in each box. Instance segmentation produces more refined image segmentation than semantic segmentation.

Generative adversarial networks (GANs) have been employed in several segmentation tasks that help the generator to produce more authentic images closer to the training data and dual adversarial training scheme in a conventional segmentation network is employed [41].

Transfer learning, a machine learning technique where a model trained on one task is re-explored on a second related task. Transfer learning is popular in deep learning due to the enormous resources required to train deep learning models both in terms of the large challenging datasets on which deep learning models are trained and the necessary computing power [42].

Data pre-processing and post-processing also play important roles [11, 43, 44].

5.2.1.1.3 Quantitative evaluation

Quantitative evaluation of the accuracy of the delineations remains a controversial area. The main controversy is the lack of consensus on the gold standard, considering the significant variations among experts as described in earlier sections. However, a number of quantitative metrics have been adopted for the evaluation of the consistency of the segmentations.

The quantitative metrics utilised include from 1D-distance, 2D-surface and 3D-volume metrics [8, 35, 45–47].

The 3D metrics are the standard volume coefficient and its variations. The standard volume coefficient, the Dice coefficient (F1 score, DC), is defined as the overlap volumes as a percentage of the union of the volumes, 2(A∩B)/A∪B. Variations of the volumetric coefficient, include: sensitivity, true positive (TPR), specificity, true negative (TNR), positive predictive value (PPV), etc.

The 2D metrics include a number of variations of the surface coefficient (SC), surface overlap (sDC) and surface positive predictive value (inclusion, sPPV), etc.

Specifically, DC sometimes referred to as DSC, is defined as,

$$\mathrm{DSC} = \frac{2\,|X \cap Y|}{|X| + |Y|},$$

where $|X|$ and $|Y|$ are the cardinality of X and Y, respectively. DSC ranges between 0 and 1, where a larger value denotes a stronger similarity. DSC = 1 when the two sets are identical.

The Jaccard coefficient or Jaccard similarity coefficient is a statistic used to quantify the similarity and diversity of samples [48]. It is defined as the intersection of samples divided by their union.

$$J(X, Y) = \frac{|X \cap Y|}{|X \cup Y|} = \frac{|X \cap Y|}{|X| + |Y| - |X \cap Y|}$$

Notably, when X and Y are empty, $J(X, Y)$ is defined as 1. The Jaccard coefficient ranges between 0 and 1. A higher $J(X, Y)$ value denotes a stronger sample similarity. Trivially, $J(X, Y) = 1$ when the two sets are equal.

The relationship between the Jaccard coefficient and DSC can be expressed as follows:

$$J(X, Y) = \frac{|X \cap Y|}{|X \cup Y|} = \frac{2\,|X \cap Y|}{2(|X| + |Y| - |X \cap Y|)} = \frac{\dfrac{2\,|X \cap Y|}{|X| + |Y|}}{2 - \dfrac{2\,|X \cap Y|}{|X| + |Y|}} = \frac{\mathrm{DICE}}{2 - \mathrm{DICE}}$$

Alternatively,

$$\mathrm{DICE} = \frac{2J(X, Y)}{1 + J(X, Y)}$$

The Jaccard coefficient and DSC produce the same rank and order to segmentation results. Therefore, either one can be selected during evaluation.

Distance metrics, reported in millimeters (mm), include variations of the Housdorff distance and average surface distance, both in signed and absolute distances.

The Hausdorff distance (HD) measures how far two subsets of a metric space are from each other. In other words, it is the greatest of all the distances from a point in one set to the closest point in the other set. Its variations include maximum distance to agreement (DTAmax), 95-percentile Hausdorff distance (HD95), slice-wise Hausdorff distance (HDsw).

HD is defined as,

$$\mathrm{HD}(X,\ Y) = \max(h(X,\ Y),\ h(Y,\ X))$$

$h(X,\ Y)$ is defined as follows:

$$h(X,\ Y) = \max_{x\in X}\min_{y\in Y}\ \|x - y\|,$$

where $\|x - y\|$ is a metric, such as Euclidean distance.

A smaller HD value denotes stronger repeatability [49]. However, HD is a maximum value. Therefore, it is extremely sensitive to extremes. HD_95 (maximum value within a 95% interval) can be used to mitigate the effects of individual singularities.

AVD, which is the average HD of all points in a set, is a more stable and less sensitive HD. It is expressed as follows:

$$\mathrm{AVD}(X, Y) = \max(d(X, Y),\ d(Y,\ X))$$

$d(x,\ y)$ is defined by

$$d(X,\ Y) = \frac{1}{N}\sum_{x\in X}\min_{y\in Y}\ \|x - y\|$$

where $\|x - y\|$ is a metric, such as Euclidean distance [49].

Variations of the average surface distance (ASD) include average symmetric surface distance (ASSD), average surface distance, maximum (ASDmax), average surface distance, mid-value (ASDmid) average distance to agreement (DTAavg).

Intrinsic limitations (data quantity; data quality)

The ultimate achievable accuracy is limited by the intrinsic quality of all the elements in the process, including the input, images as well as labels, algorithm limitations as well as application variations. The quality impact is process specific.

The quality of the input images is affected by image noise, artifact (e.g., from metal inserts), motion effect, as well as variations in the image acquisition processes. The examples of the variations in image acquisition include the imaging range, field of view, etc [12, 34, 50]. Tissues within a patient typically exhibit intensity nonuniformity. A predefined voxel size leads to partial volume averaging, namely, voxels may contain more than one tissue such that the voxel intensity may not be representative of either tissue class. There are also imaging modality specific challenges. While MR scans provide exquisite soft-tissue contrast, image intensities tend to vary between acquisitions due to magnetic susceptibility artifacts [18].

The uncertainty in volume delineation for the training images and labels as input poses significant constraints for the accuracy obtained. Contouring is inherently subjective. Learning algorithms are simply trained to maximize measures of similarity between their output and the examples given to them. Machine accuracy is only meaningful within the framework of these intrinsic uncertainties [34, 50, 51].

The available images' contrast and resolution contribute to the uncertainty. The delineation of the pancreas, for example, is difficult since numerous organs surround it, such as the liver, stomach, and intestines, have similar intensity distributions, making the boundary ambiguous. Parenchymal calcification, ductal dilation, steatosis, and image artifact can all affect the texture of the pancreas [52]. Another example is that coronary arteries are essentially invisible on the conventional CT images, delineation of coronary arteries may require fusing the angiographic image to CT images. The averaged 4DCT image, not accounting for cardiac or respiratory motion poses further uncertainty [53]. Modern CT technologies, such as dual energy CT, that aim to provide additional insight into the tissue's properties and/or improve contrast and resolution, may help mitigate some of the uncertainty.

The capability of the applied algorithm is another limiting factor. For example, the accuracy of the deformable registration limits the quality of the atlas-based organ segmentation. Some machine learning algorithms are affected by the class imbalance and morphological complexity [36, 50]. Neural networks also have known limitations (such as concerns of overfitting small medical imaging datasets due to their fully-connected architecture and corresponding large number of parameters). Many promising machine learning approaches for segmentation are still unexplored [10].

5.3 Implementation for clinical diseases: targets and normal structures

5.3.1 Head and neck and brain structures

For the head and neck region, extensive classic (atlas, anatomical/intensity models, etc) and state-of the-art algorithms (deep learning, 2D-3D models, e.g., U-Net and its variations, DeepMedic and its variations) are applied for the automated segmentations of organ at risk and targets [8, 18].

Multiple image modalities are utilized, including CT, MR, PET [8, 54].

The performance for OARs includes those for brachial plexus (DSC 0.3–0.77; HD91 15.4 mm), brain (DSC 0.84–0.99; HD3.6–18.4 mm), brainstem (DSC 0.64–0.93; HD 0.6–8.7 mm), optics chiasm (DSC 0.24–0.73; HD 1.0–5.8 mm), eyes (DSC 0.8–0.96; HD 0.4–5.3), cochlea (DSC 0.41–0.95; HD 0.7–1.7), esophagus (DSC 0.35–0.86; HD 1.1–35.8 mm), lacrimal glands (DSC 0.62–0.7), larynx (DSC 0.41–0.89; HD 6.2–12 mm), lens (DSC 0.35–0.88; HD 0.4–3.7 mm), mandible (DSC, 0.78–0.96; HD 1.3–10.9 mm), hippocampus (DSC 0.91), optic chiasm (DSC 0.24–0.91; HD 1.0–5.8 mm), left/right optic nerve (DSC, 0.3–0.9; 0.5–4.8 mm), oral cavity (DSC 0.78–0.93; HD 5.3–9.5 mm), left/right parotid (DSC, 0.72–0.91; HD 14.2–2.6 mm), pharyngeal constrictor muscle (DSC 0.5–0.8; HD HD91 2.8–14.7 mm), pituitary gland (DSC 0.3–0.9; HD91 3.2 mm), spinal cord/canal (DSC 0.37–0.96; HD 0.7–10.4 mm), and left/right submandibular (DSC 0.65–0.91; HD 3.2–9.7 mm), thyroid (DSC 0.57–0.92; HD 3.9–17.5 mm), temporal lobes (DSC 0184–0.93; HD91 4.7–12.5 mm) [8, 32, 55, 56].

For the target volumes, the following metrics are reported for lymph node clinical target volume (CTV): Dice similarity coefficient (DSC) and mean surface distance (MSD) for lymph node levels Ia through V (DSC 0.90; MSD 1.0 mm), Ib through V (Ib-V) (DSC, 0.90; MSD 1.0 mm), II through IV (II-IV) (DSC 0.89; MSD 1.1 mm), and retropharyngeal (RP) nodes (DSC 0.81; MSD 1.3 mm) [43] GTVs and CTVs can have DSC 0.62–0.83 [54, 57].

5.3.2 Thoracic and gastrointestinal structures

Many conventional atlas and model-based methodologies as well as deep learning based approaches are applied to the automated segmentations of thoracic organs at risk and targets, usually with single or multi-modality images [18].

The performance of these applications are reported for heart (DSC 0.90–0.96; HD/DTA 2.1–21.99 mm), left/right ventricles (DSC 0.75–0.92; DTA 1.3–2.7 mm), left/right atria (DSC 0.75–0.91; DTA 1.3–2.3 mm), superior/inferior venae cavae (0.78–0.88; DTA 0.9–2.9 mm), pulmonary artery/veins (DSC 0.73–0.88; DTA 0.8–2.3 mm), ascending aorta (0.78–0.92; DTA 0.9–1.6 mm), right coronary artery (DSC 0.36–0.64; DTA 1.5–2.4 mm), left main coronary artery (0.32–0.68; DTA 0.6–2.0 mm), left anterior descending coronary artery (DSC 0.36–0.92; DTA/HD 1.0–35.9 mm) [22, 44, 50, 53, 58].

Other organs at risk include esophagus (DSC 0.6–0.75; HD 3.0–12.0 mm), liver (DSC 0.87–0.99; HD95 0.7–6.3 mm), lungs (DSC 0.95–0.98; HD 1.0–11 mm), spinal cord (DSC 0.67–0.98; HD 2–11 mm), thyroid (DSC 0.70–8.85; 2–5 mm) [17, 22, 34, 37, 59, 60].

The target evaluations include those for breast CTVs (DSC 0.75–0.93; HD 3.0–22.0 mm), axillary CTVs (DSC 0.5–0.85; HD 3–15 mm), internal mammary nodes (DSC 0.5–0.8; HD 2–12 mm), supraclavicular lymph nodes (DSC 0.6–0.83; HD 3–15 mm) [22].

2–3D and variations of CNN are used to improve the performance of organ at risk for large bowel (DSC 0.84–0.96; HD95 2.5–15 mm), small bowel (DSC 0.62–0.93; HD95 2.8–29 mm), duodenum (DSC 0.65–0.96; HD95 2.2–9.8 mm), left/right kidney (DSC 0.83–0.98; HD95 0.4–7.4 mm), stomach (DSC 0.80–0.97; HD95 2.0–40.0 mm), pancreas (DSC 0.82–0.9) [34, 37, 52].

5.3.3 Pelvic structures

State-of the-art deep learning methodologies are applied for the automated structure segmentations of the organ at risk and targets in the pelvic region [18].

The performance for the organ at risk is reported for bladder (DSC 0.91–0.97; DTA/HD95 1.1–4.1 mm), bowel bag (DSC 0.82–0.85; HD95 4.4–5.6 mm), left/right femoral head (DSC 0.88–0.93; HD95 1.3–1.5 mm), small intestine (DSC 0.67–0.76), bone marrow (DSC 0.85; HD95 2.0–2.2 mm), rectum (DSC 0.65–0.86; DTA/HD95 2.7–6.0 mm) [11, 17, 37, 61].

The target performance is shown as for cervical cancer target (DSC 0.83–0.86; HD95 5.3–6.7 mm) [17], for prostate target with ultrasound (DSC 0.93–0.95; HD 2.4–4.4 mm) [35], for rectal cancer target with CT or MR images (DSC 0.73–0.94; HD 8.6–13.9 mm) [61, 62].

5.4 Best practice implementation of AI driven delineation

AI based automated segmentation has not achieved widespread adoption due to the impeding obstacles. One of the major obstacles is the insufficient supply of high-quality data. The data is needed to create effective AI tools. The bias in the data as well as other limitations affect the safety and efficacy for some populations of patients. Variations among institutions require the comprehensiveness of the input dataset that should include broad representations. The 'black box' nature of some of the AI tools makes it difficult to determine when the tool is functioning appropriately. Design and execution of a thorough clinical testing process is crucial. The ethical and regulatory concerns of the AI tools further impedes the innovation and adaptation [63].

In order to address these concerns, we need to build or extend ways for acquiring high-quality data. It is critical to promote population-representative data that is accessible, standardized, and of high quality. To assure accuracy across all populations and to attain the performance levels required for scaling success, healthcare AI should be trained and verified using population-representative data. Electronic health records and the exponential growth of consumer health data have resulted in a data-rich healthcare ecosystem. We need to address concerns with data quality, sufficient permission, interoperability, and the magnitude of data transfers.

We should encourage the establishment of standards for creating, deploying, and utilizing AI systems; utilize frameworks and best practices for machine learning in healthcare systems, human factors, and implementation science to overcome the operationalization problems associated with healthcare AI; and create and implement relevant educational and training initiatives to support healthcare AI.

We need to encourage developer–healthcare professional collaboration and establish/clarify suitable regulatory oversight processes. It is advisable to include developers of artificial intelligence, users, patients, and their families in conversations regarding suitable policy, regulatory, and legislative solutions; contextualizing the discourse around openness and trust entails acknowledging the existence of disparate requirements; prioritize ethical, egalitarian, and inclusive healthcare artificial intelligence while tackling implicit and explicit bias; regulate and legislate to strike a balance between innovation and safety and to foster trust [36, 63].

Quality assurance strategies

It is critical to construct a complete quality assurance program as part of the process of developing, establishing, and employing standards for AI systems. The quality assurance process should involve proper system commissioning, routine procedure maintenance, and patient-specific verification of auto-segmentation.

The commissioning process involves testing of the functions of a given piece of software and documentation of its different capabilities. The most obvious test for segmentation software is an evaluation of the accuracy of the segmentation, probably by comparison with manually drawn contours using overlap and distance metrics. The quantitative measurements have been discussed previously, which may also include the dose differences caused by contour discrepancies or defects in contours. Quantitative evaluations may incorporate variables such as inter-observer variability and time savings. Additionally, qualitative measurements might be used. For example, blinded head-to-head comparisons might be conducted using a modified Turing test methodology [42, 49], with auto-contoured OARs or targets being scored as 'pass' or 'fail'; or a graded subjective appraisal of the auto-segmentation model's quality [43].

The commissioning procedure should include comprehensive testing using patient data from specific institutions to confirm that the program performs as expected throughout their variety of image types, patient anatomy, and so on. It is critical to incorporate end-to-end testing to verify the data transmission and conversion processes are robust. The program should be deployed with adequate documentation outlining its capabilities and limitations.

If the AI model is developed in-house, a separate training/validation procedure is necessary. Generally, training a model requires a substantial quantity of data, preferably of good quality and annotated, that adheres to clinical guidelines and (imaging) protocols. The data should be scrutinized to ensure that it represents the patient group and clinical practice under consideration. Tumour segmentation models often require more patient data than OAR models, as tumour shapes and locations are more variable in comparison to normal anatomy. At the moment, state-of-the-art CNN-based contouring models generally include over 100 patients [40, 42]. However, it has been demonstrated that models of 50–100 patients can segment OARs with good precision [36, 38]. Typically, validation and test sets consist of roughly 20 individuals [43]. A minimum of ten patients is recommended, but this number should be raised if there is significant fluctuation in the outcome [44, 45]. The model is validated using both quantitative and qualitative analysis on a subset of data, referred to as the validation set. This collection should be representative of the clinical data to which the model will be applied. This is an iterative procedure in which model updates are made to increase performance.

For models that were not built in-house, necessary documentation includes FDA/CE certification and a vendor report outlining the model's performance. It is strongly suggested that clear information on the model's intended purpose and limitations, the description of the training and validation sets, the employed standards and the overall validation methodology are included. The vendor should give an annual accuracy evaluation process that details the annual method that the client should follow. An independent evaluation of the model's ultimate performance includes an examination of the model's robustness and a characterization of its applicability. The validation method is comparable to that of in-house built models, although slightly different. The dataset selection should encompass clinical variations, and both quantitative and qualitative assessment measures are to be used. No model alteration should be attempted to improve performance based on these unique patient circumstances. Any changes should be treated as a new version of the software.

Routine maintenance is required on an individual basis for each patient. Before any segmentation is used in a treatment plan, it should be thoroughly examined and authorized. The benefits of peer review evaluation via quality assurance contouring rounds may help assure the radiation treatment's overall safety. Automatic quality assurance of auto-segmentations may be used as a supplement to peer review or as a technique for identifying outliers. To be employed as a second peer review, the two algorithms must be completely independent.

For routine model validation, establishing a quality management program is recommended primarily to monitor for unintentional model modification, to verify that the model remains valid following a (minor) software update, and to detect and evaluate changes in the workflow (e.g., changes in imaging device, protocol, or immobilization). At the time of commissioning, a reference dataset representing clinical practice should be chosen for this purpose. The reference dataset should be re-examined for clinical representation and should include patient images acquired using the modified process. Clinical personnel should assess the model output for this new test set. Recommissioning the model may be necessary. Predictions should be made on a regular basis and compared to the original predictions (end-to-end performance) to ensure the model's consistency. Instances in which the model performed sub-optimally should be gathered to determine the model's limits, to track trends, and to permit future model changes to enhance performance for such patient cases.

To guarantee safety and clinical relevance, a specialized multidisciplinary team with necessary competence (e.g., physician, physicist, RTT, and IT professional) should be developed. This team should have a broad grasp of AI/ML/DL and a grasp of the specific model and should advise users and give training and instruction on the proper usage and interpretation of the model output. A feedback mechanism is critical to ensuring the safety and quality of care as clinical practice evolves. Prior to implementing any model, it is strongly suggested to do a risk analysis by examining the hazards. A well-known technique is failure mode and effect analysis (FMEA) [20, 22–24] or risk analysis matrices [25], which entails a brainstorming session on possible hazards involving representatives from all disciplines involved in the model's implementation and usage. Risk classification for AI tools will be impacted by the model's user control and interpretability, the degree to which humans are involved in the (QA) workflow, and the existence of safety barriers. In the event of failure or misbehaviour, other models or separate tools for the intended application should be considered [18, 64].

Education and training

The insufficiency of education and training is one of the key obstacles to widespread use of AI in medicine. However, public opinion and involvement in artificial intelligence in medicine have been improving. In June 2019, the American Medical Association established a policy integrating training in AI augmentation. The applications of artificial intelligence in radiation oncology span the disciplines of medical physicists and radiation oncologists. Certain applications, such as automated segmentation and treatment planning, will be verifiable by humans. Other applications, such as survival prognosis, decision assistance, and genomics-based treatment planning, are not human verifiable at the individual level and will thus need rigorous model construction and validation. As applied research in these areas expands in radiation oncology, a corresponding increase in education is required to develop and evaluate trustworthy AI models for clinical use.

The NCI Workshop on AI in Radiation Oncology's Training and Education Working Group (Shady Grove, MD, April 4–5, 2019) proposes an overarching action plan for radiation therapy-specific AI training comprised of various action items.

Action 1: Increase public understanding and promote appropriate use of artificial intelligence.

We should educate students on the critical nature of ethics, disparities, biases, and fairness in AI.

Implementation of a practical didactic curriculum as a second action.

Curricula must be interdisciplinary and include researchers and implementers of AI, healthcare system leadership, frontline clinical teams, ethicists, humanists, patients, and caregivers. Each group adds vital views, requirements, and expertise to the table. The curriculum should take into account the demands of medical physicists, radiation oncologists, and data scientists, as well as their individual responsibilities in the process. The program should include the following topics: 1. responsible use of AI, bias, and disparities; 2. methodology: fundamentals of data science; 3. interpreting data and models; 4. practical experience and applications; 5. data-sharing: logistical and cultural considerations.

We should require a residency curriculum to include training in artificial intelligence, big data, data privacy, and data science, and emphasize the significance of establishing a data-sharing culture via education and exposure. Data science programs should be expanded to incorporate instruction on how including diverse development teams may increase the utility and effect of AI, as well as enhance understanding of issues such as ethics, equality, inclusiveness, and unintended consequences.

Create publicly available materials as a third action.

We should establish a centralized, public repository of resources (seminal white papers, webinars, video lectures, hackathons, datasets, and code, among others); develop and disseminate radiation-specific training tools to all institutions in order to democratize access and ensure training quality; leverage trainee crowdsourcing efforts to annotate datasets for research and use annotated datasets for education.

Accelerate educational and funding opportunities.

We should utilize the AACR, ESTRO, and other organizations' workshop format for rapid learning opportunities; utilize corporate funding and interest in research via AI fellowships and tutorial workshops; identify relevant research funds for trainees and new investigators [36, 65].

5.5 Future developments and outlook

Although the future is difficult to foresee, when applied to radiation oncology imaging data, AI is anticipated to have transformational potential in the coming years. While it is natural to see the future through the prism of existing knowledge, we must expect that circumstances and capacities will likely grow much beyond their current state [66].

We lack adequate tools for reasoning about unexpected events, in part because these abilities need a causal understanding of how the Universe works. That is precisely where artificial intelligence now falls short. They modified certain aspects of the radiation oncology workflow, but they were unable to replace the complete process, and the modified components need refinement. If a physician is unable to use these technologies, they will lag behind others who can, but the tools will not completely replace the profession. AI solutions have the potential to significantly augment a clinician's capacity to care for patients [67, 68].

Significant progress is being made in areas that pose significant barriers to the widespread use of AI. The quality and quantity of data available for AI applications are increasing. The algorithms are designed to account for demographic differences between institutions. Interpretability is a feature of machine learning approaches. Data standards are being created, as well as guidelines for the creation, deployment, and use of AI systems. Policies and laws address security and privacy. However, a big concern is a shortage of people with both biomedical knowledge and algorithm-building proficiency. Substantial effort is required to resolve these obstacles in order to fully realize AI's promise [36, 63, 69, 70].

References

[1] Bentzen S M *et al* 2010 Quantitative analyses of normal tissue effects in the clinic (QUANTEC): an introduction to the scientific issues *Int. J. Radiat. Oncol. Biol. Phys.* **76**

[2] Milano M T *et al* 2021 Single-and multi-fraction stereotactic radiosurgery dose tolerances of the optic pathways *Int. J. Radiat. Oncol. Biol. Phys.* **110** 87–99

[3] Mir R *et al* 2020 Organ at risk delineation for radiation therapy clinical trials: Global Harmonization Group consensus guidelines *Radiother. Oncol.* **150** 30–9

[4] Mayo C S *et al* 2017 AAPM TG-263: standardizing nomenclatures in radiation oncology *Int. J. Radiat. Oncol. Biol. Phys.* **100** 1057–66

[5] Milo M L H *et al* 2020 Delineation of whole heart and substructures in thoracic radiation therapy: national guidelines and contouring atlas by the Danish Multidisciplinary Cancer Groups *Radiother. Oncol.* **150** 121–27

[6] Riegel A C, Vaccarelli M, Cox B W, Chou H, Cao Y and Potters L 2019 Impact of multi-institutional prospective peer review on target and organ-at-risk delineation in radiation therapy *Practical Radiation Oncology* **9** e228–35

[7] van der Veen J, Gulyban A and Nuyts S 2019 Interobserver variability in delineation of target volumes in head and neck cancer *Radiother. Oncol.* **137** 9–15

[8] Vrtovec T, Močnik D, Strojan P, Pernuš F and Ibragimov B 2020 Auto-segmentation of organs at risk for head and neck radiotherapy planning: from atlas-based to deep learning methods *Med. Phys.* **47** e929–50

[9] Roach D *et al* 2019 Multi-observer contouring of male pelvic anatomy: highly variable agreement across conventional and emerging structures of interest *J. Med. Imag. Radiat. Oncol.* **63** 264–71

[10] Macomber M W *et al* 2018 Autosegmentation of prostate anatomy for radiation treatment planning using deep decision forests of radiomic features *Phys. Med. Biol.* **63** 0–11
[11] Zabel W J *et al* 2021 Clinical evaluation of deep learning and atlas-based auto-contouring of bladder and rectum for prostate radiation therapy *Pract. Radiat. Oncol.* **11** e80–9
[12] Kosmin M *et al* 2019 Rapid advances in auto-segmentation of organs at risk and target volumes in head and neck cancer *Radiother. Oncol.* **135** 130–40
[13] Aliotta E, Nourzadeh H and Siebers J 2019 Quantifying the dosimetric impact of organ-at-risk delineation variability in head and neck radiation therapy in the context of patient setup uncertainty *Phys. Med. Biol.* **64** 0–14
[14] Ohri N, Shen X, Dicker A P, Doyle L A, Harrison A S and Showalter T N 2013 Radiotherapy protocol deviations and clinical outcomes: a meta-analysis of cooperative group clinical trials *J. Natl Cancer Inst.* **105** 387–93
[15] Peters L J *et al* 2010 Critical impact of radiotherapy protocol compliance and quality in the treatment of advanced head and neck cancer: results from TROG 02.02 *J. Clin. Oncol. Off. J. Am. Soc. Clin. Oncol.* **28** 2996–3001
[16] Rouard N *et al* 2019 Intensity-modulated radiation therapy of anal squamous cell carcinoma: relationship between delineation quality and regional recurrence *Radiother. Oncol.* **131** 93–100
[17] Liu Z *et al* 2020 Development and validation of a deep learning algorithm for auto-delineation of clinical target volume and organs at risk in cervical cancer radiotherapy *Radiother. Oncol.* **153** 172–79
[18] Cardenas C E, Yang J, Anderson B M, Court L E and Brock K B 2019 Advances in auto-segmentation *Semin. Radiat. Oncol.* **29** 185–97
[19] Nigam V, Luthra S and Bhatnagar S 2010 A comparative study of thresholding techniques for image denoising, *2010 Int. Conf. on Computer and Communication Technology, ICCCT-2010* 173–6
[20] Mueller M, Segl K and Kaufmann H 2004 Edge- and region-based segmentation technique for the extraction of large, man-made objects in high-resolution satellite imagery *Pattern Recognit.* **37** 1619–628
[21] Al-amri S S, Kalyankar N V and KhamitkarS D 2010 Image segmentation by using edge detection *Int. J. Comput. Scie. Eng.* **2** 804–07
[22] Choi M S *et al* 2020 Clinical evaluation of atlas- and deep learning-based automatic segmentation of multiple organs and clinical target volumes for breast cancer *Radiother. Oncol.* **153** 139–45
[23] Van Ginneken B, Frangi A F, Staal J J, Ter Haar Romeny B M and Viergever M A 2002 Active shape model segmentation with optimal features, *IEEE Trans. Med. Imaging* **21** 924–33
[24] Shen C, Nguyen D, Zhou Z, Jiang S B, Dong B and Jia X 2020 An introduction to deep learning in medical physics: advantages, potential, and challenges, *Phys. Med. Biol.* **65** 0–29
[25] Mcculloch W S and Pitts W 1943 A logical calculus of the ideas immanent in nervous activity *Bull. Math. Biophys.* **5** 115–33
[26] LeCun Y, Boser B, Denker J, Henderson D, Howard R, Hubbard W and Jackel L 1989 Handwritten digit recognition with a back-propagation network *Advances in Neural Information Processing Systems 2 (NIPS 1989)*
[27] Krizhevsky A, Sutskever I and Hinton G E 2017 ImageNet classification with deep convolutional neural networks *Commun. ACM* **60** 84–90

[28] Simonyan K and Zisserman A 2014 Very deep convolutional networks for large-scale image recognition arXiv:1409.1556
[29] Szegedy C *et al* Oct. 2015 Going deeper with convolutions, *Proc. of the IEEE Computer Society Conf. on Computer Vision and Pattern Recognition* vol 7 1–9
[30] Navab N, Hornegger J, Wells W M and Frangi A F 2015 Medical image computing and computer-assisted intervention—*MICCAI 2015: 18th Int. Conf. Munich, Germany, October 5–9, 2015 proceedings, part III*, (Lecture Notes in Computer Science (including subseries Lecture Notes in Artificial Intelligence and Lecture Notes in Bioinformatics) vol 9351) (Cham: Springer) pp 12–20
[31] Milletari F, Navab N and Ahmadi S A 2016 V-Net: fully convolutional neural networks for volumetric medical image segmentation *Proc. 2016 4th Int. Conf. on 3D Vision, 3DV 2016* 565–71
[32] Liu Y *et al* 2020 Head and neck multi-organ auto-segmentation on CT images aided by synthetic MRI *Med. Phys.* **47** 4294–302
[33] Feng F, Ashton-Miller J A, DeLancey J O L and Luo J 2020 Convolutional neural network-based pelvic floor structure segmentation using magnetic resonance imaging in pelvic organ prolapse *Med. Phys.* **47** 4281–293
[34] Liu Y *et al* 2020 CT-based multi-organ segmentation using a 3D self-attention U-net network for pancreatic radiotherapy *Med. Phys.* **47** 4316–324
[35] Orlando N, Gillies D J, Gyacskov I, Romagnoli C, D'Souza D and Fenster A 2020 Automatic prostate segmentation using deep learning on clinically diverse 3D transrectal ultrasound images *Med. Phys.* **47** 2413–426
[36] Tong N, Gou S, Niu T, Yang S and Sheng K 2020 Self-paced densenet with boundary constraint for automated multi-organ segmentation on abdominal CT images *Phys. Med. Biol.* **65**
[37] Weston A D *et al* 2020 Complete abdomen and pelvis segmentation using U-net variant architecture *Med. Phys.* **47** 5609–618
[38] Mak R H *et al* 2019 Use of crowd innovation to develop an artificial intelligence-based solution for radiation therapy targeting *JAMA Oncol.* **5** 654–61
[39] Simonyan K and Zisserman A 2015 Very deep convolutional networks for large-scale image recognition, *3rd Int. Conf. on Learning Representations, ICLR 2015—Conf. Track Proc.* 1–4
[40] He K, Gkioxari G, Dollár P and Girshick R 2020 Mask R-CNN *IEEE Trans. Pattern Anal. Mach. Intell.* **42** 386–97
[41] Li M, Lian F and Guo S 2020 Pancreas segmentation based on an adversarial model under two-tier constraints *Phys. Med. Biol.* **65** 0–12
[42] Yosinski J, Clune J, Bengio Y and Lipson H 2014 How transferable are features in deep neural networks? *Adv. Neur. Inform. Proc. Syst.* **4** 3320–328
[43] Cardenas C E *et al* 2021 Generating high-quality lymph node clinical target volumes for head and neck cancer radiation therapy using a fully automated deep learning-based approach *Int. J. Radiat. Oncol. Biol. Phys.* **109** 801–12
[44] Haq R, Hotca A, Apte A, Rimner A, Deasy J O and Thor M 2020 Cardio-pulmonary substructure segmentation of radiotherapy computed tomography images using convolutional neural networks for clinical outcomes analysis *Phys. Imag. Radiat. Oncol.* **14** 61–6
[45] Zou K H *et al* 2004 Statistical validation of image segmentation quality based on a spatial overlap index *Acad. Radiol.* **11** 178–89
[46] Zhu J *et al* 2020 Evaluation of automatic segmentation model with dosimetric metrics for radiotherapy of esophageal cancer *Front. Oncol.* **10** 1–9

[47] Vaassen F *et al* 2020 Evaluation of measures for assessing time-saving of automatic organ-at-risk segmentation in radiotherapy *Phys. Imag. Radiat. Oncol.* **13** 1–6
[48] Eelbode T *et al* 2020 Optimization for medical image segmentation: theory and practice when evaluating with dice score or Jaccard index *IEEE Trans. Med. Imaging* **39** 3679–90
[49] Taha A A and Hanbury A 2015 Metrics for evaluating 3D medical image segmentation: analysis, selection, and tool *BMC Med. Imaging* **15** 29
[50] Finnegan R *et al* 2021 Validation of a new open-source method for automatic delineation and dose assessment of the heart and LADCA in breast radiotherapy with simultaneous uncertainty estimation *Phys. Med. Biol.* **66** 035014
[51] Jarrett D, Stride E, Vallis K and Gooding M J 2019 Applications and limitations of machine learning in radiation oncology *Br. J. Radiol.* **92** 20190001
[52] Zheng H, Qian L, Qin Y, Gu Y and Yang J 2020 Improving the slice interaction of 2.5D CNN for automatic pancreas segmentation *Med. Phys.* **47** 5543–554
[53] Luo Y *et al* 2019 Automatic segmentation of cardiac substructures from noncontrast CT images: accurate enough for dosimetric analysis? *Acta Oncol.* **58** 81–7
[54] Guo Z, Guo N, Gong K, Zhong S and Li Q 2019 Gross tumor volume segmentation for head and neck cancer radiotherapy using deep dense multi-modality network *Phys. Med. Biol.* **64** 0–14
[55] van Rooij W, Dahele M, Ribeiro Brandao H, Delaney A R, Slotman B J and Verbakel W F 2019 Deep learning-based delineation of head and neck organs at risk: geometric and dosimetric evaluation *Int. J. Radiat. Oncol. Biol. Phys.* **104** 677–84
[56] Chen H *et al* 2019 A recursive ensemble organ segmentation (REOS) framework: application in brain radiotherapy *Phys. Med. Biol.* **64** 0–12
[57] Men K *et al* 2017 Deep deconvolutional neural network for target segmentation of nasopharyngeal cancer in planning computed tomography images *Front. Oncol.* **7** 315
[58] Morris E D, Ghanem A I, Dong M, Pantelic M V, Walker E M and Glide-Hurst C K 2020 Cardiac substructure segmentation with deep learning for improved cardiac sparing, *Med. Phys.* **47** 576–86
[59] Men K, Geng H, Biswas T, Liao Z and Xiao Y 2020 Automated quality assurance of OAR contouring for lung cancer based on segmentation with deep active learning *Front. Oncol.* **10** 986
[60] Zhu J, Zhang J, Qiu B, Liu Y, Liu X and Chen L 2019 Comparison of the automatic segmentation of multiple organs at risk in CT images of lung cancer between deep convolutional neural network-based and atlas-based techniques *Acta Oncol.* **58** 257–64
[61] Song Y *et al* 2020 Automatic delineation of the clinical target volume and organs at risk by deep learning for rectal cancer postoperative radiotherapy *Radiother. Oncol.* **145** 186–92
[62] Wang M *et al* 2019 Full convolutional network based multiple side-output fusion architecture for the segmentation of rectal tumors in magnetic resonance images: a multi-vendor study *Med. Phys.* **46** 2659–668
[63] Rubin R 2021 Obstacles to implementing AI tools in health care *JAMA* **325** 333
[64] Vandewinckele L *et al* 2020 Overview of artificial intelligence-based applications in radiotherapy: recommendations for implementation and quality assurance *Radiother. Oncol.* **153** 55–66
[65] Kang J *et al* 2021 National cancer institute workshop on artificial intelligence in radiation oncology: training the next generation *Practical Radiation Oncology* **11** 74–83
[66] Thompson R F *et al* 2018 Artificial intelligence in radiation oncology imaging *Int. J. Radiat. Oncol. Biol. Phys.* **102** 1159–161

[67] Desai A N 2021 Artificial intelligence: promise, pitfalls, and perspective *JAMA* **323** 244–9
[68] Coiera E 2019 On algorithms, machines, and medicine *Lancet Oncol.* **20** 166–67
[69] Maddox T M, Rumsfeld J S and Payne P R O 2019 Questions for artificial intelligence in health care *JAMA* **321** 31–2
[70] Boucher P 2019 How artificial intelligence works *STOA | Panel for the Future of Science and Technology* **3** 10
[71] Ronneberger O, Fischer P, Brox T 2015 U-Net: convolutional networks for biomedical image segmentation *Medical Image Computing and Computer-Assisted Intervention—* MICCAI 2015 ed N Navab, J Hornegger, W Wells and A Frangi (Lecture Notes in Computer Science, vol 9351) (Cham: Springer)
[72] He K et al 2017 Mask *r*-cnn *Proc. of the IEEE Int. Conf. on Computer Vision.* 2017 2961–9 https://openaccess.thecvf.com/content_ICCV_2017/papers/He_Mask_R-CNN_ICCV_2017_paper.pdf

Chapter 6

Automated treatment planning

Charles Huang and Lei Xing

In this chapter we provide a brief overview of automated treatment planning methods. We introduce the three main categories of methods (i.e., KBP, PBP, and MCO), summarizing their advantages and limitations. The field of automated treatment planning has been growing rapidly in recent years, and we look forward to continued developments in the field.

6.1 Goals and motivations of treatment planning

Treatment planning is the process of determining various treatment parameters (i.e., beam fluences, leaf positions, aperture weights, etc) that are critical to management of a patient's disease [1]. We can conceptualize the clinical objective of treatment planning as the intent to treat diseased tissue while the minimizing dose to healthy organs. Traditionally, the treatment planning process has been performed by a team of personnel, which consists of radiation oncologists, radiation therapists, medical physicists, and dosimetrists.

There are two main types of radiation therapy that utilize treatment planning: external beam radiation therapy (EBRT) and internal radiation therapy (i.e., brachytherapy). In the treatment planning process, we begin by collecting medical images for the patient (e.g., CT, MRI, or PET scans). From these medical images, the target volumes and organs-at-risk (OARs) can then be delineated. Following guidelines, such as those from the International Commission on Radiation Units and Measurements (ICRU), we can perform contouring for structures like the planning target volume (PTV), clinical target volume (CTV), and gross tumor volume (GTV). Similarly, volumes of interest for OARs can be segmented manually or automatically. Computed tomography (CT) is the primary imaging modality used for treatment planning. Magnetic resonance imaging (MRI) is also commonly used and can be especially useful in cases that require better soft tissue contrast. Positron emission tomography (PET) may also be used for staging disease and

doi:10.1088/978-0-7503-3339-9ch6

assessing the target volume, as these images complement the anatomical information from CT and MRI.

Conventional treatment planning can be formulated as an inverse problem. Following this formulation, we first determine input criteria in the form of objectives and constraints on the target and OARs. Optimization is then performed to find a treatment plan configuration (i.e., beam fluences, aperture shape, etc) that satisfies the given input criteria. Evaluation of these treatment plan solutions typically incorporates visualizations of the dose distribution, dose-volume histogram (DVH), and isodose lines, as well as various plan metrics (e.g., conformity index, homogeneity index, etc).

Treatment planning, however, is a multi-objective problem with potentially many conflicting objectives. As such, there is no single treatment plan solution that can be globally optimal for all considered objectives. Instead, we might consider efficient plans as those that are Pareto optimal, where improvements in one objective can only be made at the expense of other objectives.

Inverse planning optimization alone may not necessarily guarantee that a treatment plan solution is clinically acceptable. To improve the acceptability of produced plans, human planners traditionally perform treatment planning through a manual, iterative process. In this process, planners repeatedly adjust parameters such as objective weights, reference doses, dose constraint bounds, etc, until an acceptable treatment plan solution is found. The iterative planning process is not only time-consuming and labor intensive (i.e., long active planning times), but the resulting plan quality highly depends on planner skill and experience [2]. Automated methods, therefore, aim to reduce active planning time and standardize plan quality, with fully automated methods requiring no active planning (figure 6.1).

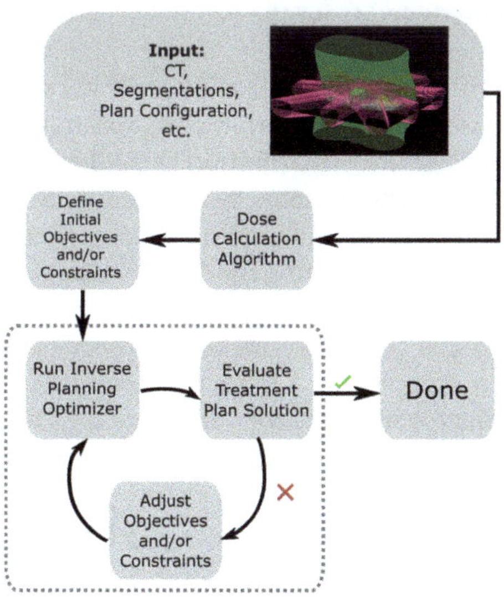

Figure 6.1. Visualization of the manual treatment planning process. Reprinted with permission from [47], copyright 2022 by Charles Huang.

6.2 Automated treatment planning overview

Manual planning, for context, has two main limitations: long active planning times and high inter-planner variability. First, the manual planning process is traditionally performed with iterative adjustments to treatment planning parameters (e.g., objective weights, reference doses, constraint bounds, etc) and requires planners to be actively involved throughout planning, which results in long active planning times. Second, evaluation of each treatment plan and judgment on when to end the iterative process are decisions left up to individual planners. The manual planning process can be conceptualized as a balancing act where exploration of all objective and constraint configurations is likely to be infeasible. For this reason, iterative manual planning does not provide any guarantees on plan acceptability and, instead, involves a trade-off between improving acceptability and spending a reasonable amount of time actively planning. Consequently, while there are many protocols and guidelines in place for quality assurance [3–5], plan quality nevertheless varies with a planner's skill and experience.

Automated treatment planning methods have been an active area of research since the inception of IMRT inverse planning [1, 6]. These automated methods generally aim to reduce active planning time and inter-planner variability [2]. We can classify automated methods using the following categories: knowledge-based planning (KBP), protocol-based planning (PBP), and multicriteria optimization (MCO) [2]. Here, we survey some of the relevant works to provide context for the benefits and drawbacks of these automated methods when used in clinical workflow.

6.3 Knowledge-based planning

KBP methods are a category of methods based on the premise that treatment planning results can be predicted from the geometric and anatomical information of a patient [7]. KBP attempts to reduce active planning times by leveraging information learned from a knowledge base of previous plans. Various approaches in KBP have been proposed that range from class solutions to predicting the DVH, and even to predicting the 3D dose distribution [2, 8]. From these predictions, a plan can then be constructed for new patients to be used as an initial guess for further manual planning or as the final accepted plan. KBP typically follows the paradigm of training a supervised machine learning model on a dataset of previously generated treatment plans. One common way to form these datasets for training is to collect and aggregate manual plans that were created as part of clinical workflow. Once data collection has been completed, a supervised model can be trained to predict treatment planning results for new patients. In figure 6.2, we provide a visualization

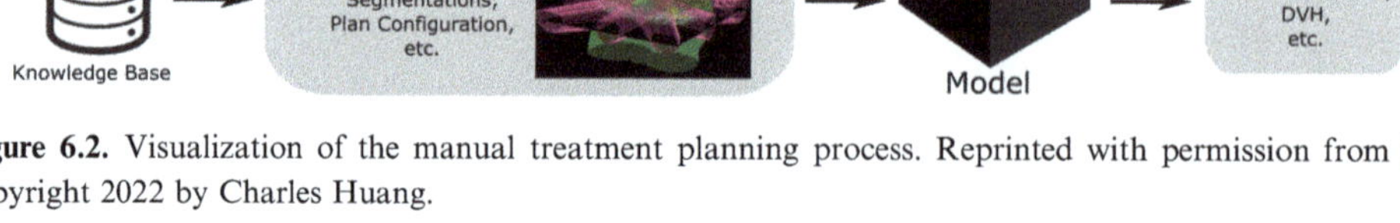

Figure 6.2. Visualization of the manual treatment planning process. Reprinted with permission from [47], copyright 2022 by Charles Huang.

of the overall workflow for supervised KBP. Given sufficient input information (as an example, we might include a patient's CT and structure segmentations), KBP models attempt to predict the voxel-wise dose distribution or the dose-volume histogram (DVH) [7, 9–12]. KBP models have also been used to predict machine parameters directly [13, 14], where additional dose mimicking steps are taken after a dose prediction in order to translate those predictions into deliverable plans. Current dose mimicking methods typically utilize a simple L2-norm penalty when performing dose mimicking, which may not be entirely appropriate given that treatment planning is a multicriteria optimization problem. Interestingly, it is also possible to perform KBP by eliminating the dose prediction step and predicting machine parameters directly. However, current methods for these end-to-end predictions have not yet been able to produce satisfactory treatment plans [15].

The main advantage of KBP methods is fast computation times during model deployment. KBP methods typically involve the use of learning-based methods (i.e., supervised learning). Following this type of approach, we form a database of previously generated treatment plans to serve as the ground truth for training a model. Often, these ground truth treatment plans are a collection of manual plans used as part of research or clinical workflow. While the training process of these KBP models may be computationally expensive, deployment of a trained model on future plans is exceedingly fast, which represents one key advantage of KBP methods.

The main disadvantages of current KBP methods are the lack of interpretability and performance guarantees. KBP methods typically involve training 'black-box' models on a database of treatment plans. Improving the interpretability of these models has been an ongoing area of research [16–20], as interpretability is critically important for troubleshooting, safety, integration in clinical workflow, and so forth. Previous works provide empirical evidence that KBP models can perform reasonably well, often matching the performance of manual plans created in the clinic [7, 9, 10]. In cases where KBP performs poorly, however, lack of model interpretability limits the usability of KBP approaches. The second main limitation of current KBP methods is its lack of performance guarantees. As KBP models are typically trained using supervised learning with manual plans as the ground truth, ensuring that the model predictions are efficient (i.e., Pareto optimal) proves difficult, especially when considering that the manual ground truth treatment plans may not be efficient either. In other words, KBP methods often make no guarantees about the efficiency of produced plans and, instead, only attempt to mimic the ground truth data used in training. Combined, these drawbacks may limit the practical usability of KBP methods in the clinic, at least in their present forms [21].

6.4 Protocol-based planning

PBP methods are a category of methods that employ rules or heuristics to mimic an experienced treatment planner performing iterative planning. Previous works have proposed various rules for adjusting treatment planning parameters (i.e., objective weights, constraint values, etc) based on advice from consulted physicians [2]. Others have followed a model-free approach, opting to use reinforcement learning to mimic human planners [22].

Specific approaches to PBP are highly varied, although they share the common goal of automating the iterative adjustments used in manual planning. On one end of the spectrum, there are PBP approaches that interface with existing treatment planning software by automating mouse cursor movement and keyboard input [23]. Other variations involve accessing the treatment planning system through scripting API [24–31]. A commercial implementation of PBP can be accessed within the Phillips Pinnacle[3] system [32, 33].

While PBP methods may offer a practical approach to automation, they also inherit some of the same limitations of manual planning. In manual planning, planners trade-off improved plan efficiency and long active planning times. PBP helps to reduce active planning times but does not directly guarantee that the produced plans are efficient. To ensure efficiency of the produced treatment plans, we instead look to the next category of automated methods: multicriteria optimization.

6.5 Multicriteria optimization

To recap, treatment planning involves optimization of multiple, potentially conflicting objectives. For nontrivial problems, no single treatment plan will optimize all considered objectives at once. To produce efficient plans, we instead attempt to explore the set of Pareto optimal treatment plans, which we subsequently refer to as the Pareto front. These Pareto optimal plans are nondominated where improvements to one objective can only be made at the expense of other objectives.

$$\begin{aligned} \min_{x} \quad & \frac{w_1}{N_{\text{ptv}}} \sum_{i \in \text{ptv}} \left(d_i - D_p\right)^2 + \frac{w_2}{N_{\text{OAR}}} \sum_{i \in \text{OAR}} d_i^2 \\ s.\,t. \quad & x \geqslant 0 \\ & w \geqslant 0 \\ & \vec{d} = \boldsymbol{D}\vec{x} \end{aligned} \tag{6.1}$$

We begin with the weighted sum method, which is directly applicable to manual planning. To start we specify nonnegative weights for each objective function being considered. Equation (6.1) provides a hypothetical example case with two objectives. Here, D_p refers to the prescription dose, d_i refers to the dose at voxel i, w refers to the nonnegative weight vector, N refers to the total number of voxels in a specific structure, and D refers to the dose-influence matrix. In the weighted sum approach, the MCO problem has been transformed into a single objective problem for a given set of importance weights. By solving the weighted sum objective for various nonnegative weight configurations, we can potentially find the Pareto front for convex problems. In the case of nonconvex problems, however, many weight configurations may collapse to similar solutions on the Pareto front, and we may be unable to find all the Pareto optimal solutions. Figure 6.3 provides a visualization of the weighted sum

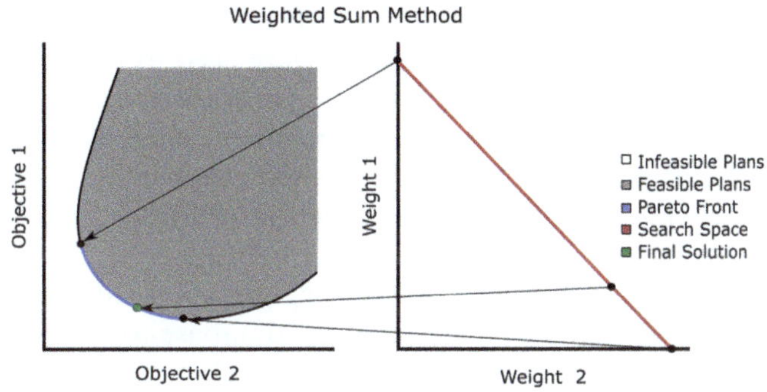

Figure 6.3. Visualization of the weighted sum method for a hypothetical case with two objectives. Copyright (2021) IEEE. Reprinted, with permission, from [44].

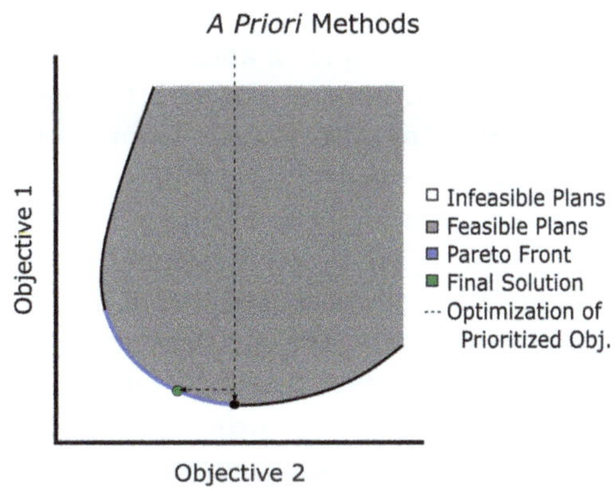

Figure 6.4. Visualization of an *a priori* method, we use the lexicographic method as an example, for a hypothetical case with two objectives. Copyright (2021) IEEE. Reprinted, with permission, from [44].

approach for a hypothetical case with two objectives. In general, MCO methods can be classified into two categories: *a priori* and *a posteriori* methods.

In *a priori* MCO, a Pareto optimal solution is found according to provided preferences. Such approaches require sufficient preference information to be provided by the planner, and some notable examples include scalarization (e.g., ϵ-constraint method, achievement scalarization, etc) [2, 34, 35], prioritized optimization [36–38], and the lexicographic method [39, 40]. Conceptually, *a priori* methods can be thought of as using provided preference information to navigate through the treatment plan solution space in search of a Pareto optimal solution. In figure 6.4, we visualize the lexicographic method for a hypothetical case with two objectives. In the lexicographic method, we begin by establishing a ranking of various objectives according to provided preference information. We then adopt an iterative approach where each objective is optimized in sequence according to the established ranking. Translating physicians' intuitions regarding ideal planning to a list of preferences, however, is no trivial task, and sometimes treatment plan solutions found from preference information may not align with planner expectations. In these cases, it is likely that the provided preference information may need to be modified.

A posteriori methods, by contrast, attempt to generate or approximate the Pareto front, creating a database of Pareto optimal treatment plans that a human planner might choose from. Previous works have proposed alternative ways to generate the Pareto front (e.g., Pareto surface generation or PGEN, simulated annealing, evolutionary algorithms, etc) [2, 41–44]. A visualization of the decision-making process in *a posteriori* methods is provided in figure 6.5. Traditionally, *a posteriori* methods delegate the selection of plans from the database to a human planner, and this selection process follows the general scheme of picking desirable plans according to their utility or clinical acceptability [43, 44]. While the selection process in *a posteriori* methods has been performed manually in the past, more recent works adopt a fully automated approach to the selection process [44, 45].

The Pareto optimal projection search (POPS) method provides one approach to fully automated MCO [44, 45]. In traditional *a posteriori* MCO approaches, we generate a database of Pareto optimal plans, and the most desirable plan from that database is manually selected by a human planner. The POPS method automates this selection process by searching the Pareto front using a provided scoring function. There are two main components of the POPS method: gradient-free search and projections using the bisection method. Figure 6.6 provides a visualization of the POPS method for a hypothetical two-dimensional case. Following the POPS method we begin by defining a search space (red line in figure 6.6) by first projecting a seed point to the feasibility boundary. We can then apply any gradient-free search method, such as the Nelder-Mead simplex search [46], where each point in the search space is projected to the feasibility boundary using the bisection method. Intuitively, we can conceptualize this method as searching the feasibility boundary (which contains the Pareto front) for the most desirable plans, just as is done in traditional *a posteriori* MCO.

MCO approaches also have various limitations. Traditional MCO approaches, for instance, are not fully automated. In *a posteriori* MCO, the decision-making

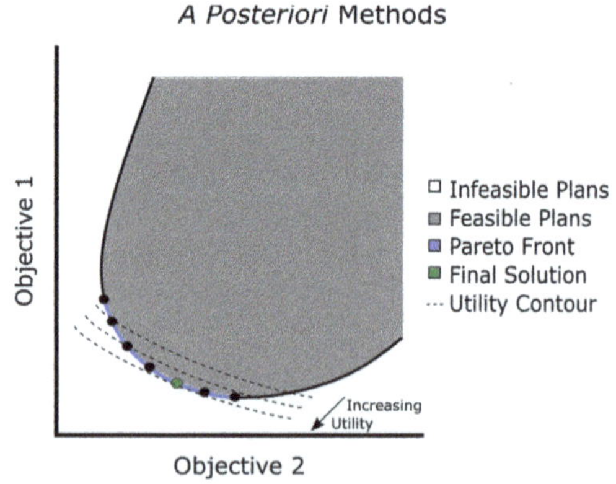

Figure 6.5. Visualization of the decision-making process in *a posteriori* methods for a hypothetical case with two objectives. Copyright (2021) IEEE. Reprinted, with permission, from [44].

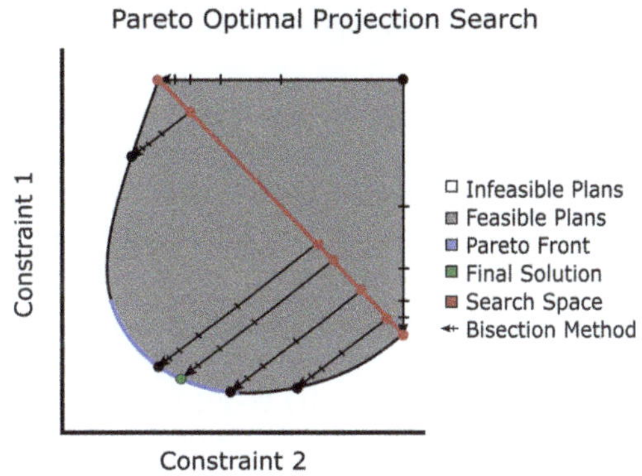

Figure 6.6. Visualization of the POPS method where the manual decision-making process in *a posteriori* MCO has been converted into a fully automated search. The POPS method consists of a gradient-free search of the defined search space (red line) and a projection of points from the search space to the feasibility boundary. Copyright (2021) IEEE. Reprinted, with permission, from [44].

process is performed by a human planner. Similarly, in *a priori* MCO, the definition of preference information is usually performed and updated manually. Fully automated MCO methods (i.e., POPS, ECHO, etc) perform the decision-making process without requiring active planning input from human planners. Instead, they remove the active planning time requirement at the expense of increased background computation time [40, 44, 45].

References

[1] Sethi A 2016 *Khan's Treatment Planning in Radiation Oncology* 4th edn ed F M Khan, J P Gibbons and P W Sperduto (Philadelphia, PA: Wolters Kluwer)

[2] Hussein M, Heijmen B J M, Verellen D and Nisbet A 2018 Automation in intensity modulated radiotherapy treatment planning—a review of recent innovations *Br. J. Radiol.* **91** 20180270

[3] Michalski J M, Moughan J, Purdy J, Bosch W, Bruner D W and Bahary J-P *et al* 2018 Effect of standard vs dose-escalated radiation therapy for patients with intermediate-risk prostate cancer: the NRG oncology RTOG 0126 randomized clinical trial *JAMA Oncol.* **4** e180039

[4] Hong T S, Moughan J, Garofalo M C, Bendell J, Berger A C and Oldenburg N B E *et al* 2015 NRG oncology radiation therapy oncology group 0822: a phase II study of preoperative chemoradiotherapy utilizing intensity modulated radiation therapy (IMRT) in combination with capecitabine and oxaliplatin for patients with locally advanced rectal cancer *Int. J. Radiat. Oncol. Biol. Phys.* **93** 29–36

[5] Lee N, Harris J, Garden A S, Straube W, Glisson B and Xia P *et al* 2009 Intensity-modulated radiation therapy with or without chemotherapy for nasopharyngeal carcinoma: radiation therapy oncology group phase II trial 0225 *J. Clin. Oncol. Off. J. Am. Soc. Clin. Oncol.* **27** 3684–90

[6] Xing L, Li J G, Donaldson S, Le Q T and Boyer A L 1999 Optimization of importance factors in inverse planning *Phys. Med. Biol.* **44** 2525–36

[7] Ge Y and Wu Q J 2019 Knowledge-based planning for intensity-modulated radiation therapy: a review of data-driven approaches *Med. Phys.* **46** 2760–75

[8] Schreibmann E and Xing L 2004 Feasibility study of beam orientation class-solutions for prostate IMRT *Med. Phys.* **31** 2863–70
[9] Ma M, Kovalchuk N, Buyyounouski M K, Xing L and Yang Y 2019 Incorporating dosimetric features into the prediction of 3D VMAT dose distributions using deep convolutional neural network *Phys. Med. Biol.* **64** 125017
[10] Fogliata A, Belosi F, Clivio A, Navarria P, Nicolini G and Scorsetti M *et al* 2014 Dec 1 On the pre-clinical validation of a commercial model-based optimisation engine: application to volumetric modulated arc therapy for patients with lung or prostate cancer *Radiother. Oncol.* **113** 385–91
[11] Korani M M, Dong P and Xing L 2016 MO-G-201-03: deep-learning based prediction of achievable dose for personalizing inverse treatment planning *Med. Phys.* **43** 3724–724
[12] Ma M, Buyyounouski M K, Vasudevan V, Xing L and Yang Y 2019 Dose distribution prediction in isodose feature-preserving voxelization domain using deep convolutional neural network *Med. Phys.* **46** 2978–87
[13] Fan J, Wang J, Chen Z, Hu C, Zhang Z and Hu W 2019 Automatic treatment planning based on three-dimensional dose distribution predicted from deep learning technique *Med. Phys.* **46** 370–81
[14] Mahmood R, Babier A, McNiven A, Diamant A and Chan T C Y 2018 Automated treatment planning in radiation therapy using generative adversarial networks ArXiv: 1807.06489
[15] Bice N, Fakhreddine M, Li R, Nguyen D, Kabat C and Myers P *et al* 2021 Latent space arc therapy optimization *Phys. Med. Biol.* **66** 215019
[16] Molnar C 2019 *Interpretable Machine Learning: A Guide for Making Black Box Models Explainable* (independently published)
[17] Barocas S, Hardt M and Narayanan A 2019 *Fairness and Machine Learning* https://fairmlbook.org/
[18] Chakraborty S, Tomsett R, Raghavendra R, Harborne D, Alzantot M and Cerutti F *et al* 2017 Interpretability of deep learning models: a survey of results *2017 IEEE SmartWorld, Ubiquitous Intelligence Computing, Advanced Trusted Computed, Scalable Computing Communications, Cloud Big Data Computing, Internet of People and Smart City Innovation (SmartWorld/SCALCOM/UIC/ATC/CBDCom/IOP/SCI)* 1–6
[19] Gilpin L H, Bau D, Yuan B Z, Bajwa A, Specter M and Kagal L 2018 Explaining explanations: an overview of interpretability of machine learning *IEEE 5th Int. Conf. on Data Science and Advanced Analytics (DSAA)* 2018 80–9
[20] Rudin C 2019 Stop explaining black box machine learning models for high stakes decisions and use interpretable models instead *Nat. Mach. Intell.* **1** 206–15
[21] Xing L, Giger M and Min J *Artificial Intelligence Medicine: Technical Basis and Clinical Applications* 1st edn (St. Louis, MO: Elsevier S&T Books) 568 pp Available from: https://elsevier.com/books/artificial-intelligence-in-medicine/xing/978-0-12–821259-2
[22] Shen C, Nguyen D, Chen L, Gonzalez Y, McBeth R and Qin N *et al* 2020 Operating a treatment planning system using a deep-reinforcement learning-based virtual treatment planner for prostate cancer intensity-modulated radiation therapy treatment planning *Med. Phys.* **47** 2329–36
[23] Tol J P, Dahele M, Peltola J, Nord J, Slotman B J and Verbakel W F A R 2015 Automatic interactive optimization for volumetric modulated arc therapy planning *Radiat. Oncol. Lond. Engl.* **10** 75

[24] Boylan C and Rowbottom C 2014 A bias-free, automated planning tool for technique comparison in radiotherapy - application to nasopharyngeal carcinoma treatments *J. Appl. Clin. Med. Phys.* **15** 4530
[25] Krayenbuehl J, Di Martino M, Guckenberger M and Andratschke N 2017 Improved plan quality with automated radiotherapy planning for whole brain with hippocampus sparing: a comparison to the RTOG 0933 trial *Radiat. Oncol. Lond. Engl.* **12** 161
[26] Zhang X, Li X, Quan E M, Pan X and Li Y 2011 A methodology for automatic intensity-modulated radiation treatment planning for lung cancer *Phys. Med. Biol.* **56** 3873–93
[27] Yan H, Yin F-F and Willett C 2007 Evaluation of an artificial intelligence guided inverse planning system: clinical case study *Radiother. Oncol. J. Eur. Soc. Ther. Radiol. Oncol.* **83** 76–85
[28] Yan H, Yin F-F, Guan H and Kim J H 2003 Fuzzy logic guided inverse treatment planning *Med. Phys.* **30** 2675–85
[29] Yan H, Yin F-F, Guan H and Kim J H 2003 AI-guided parameter optimization in inverse treatment planning *Phys. Med. Biol.* **48** 3565–80
[30] Xhaferllari I, Wong E, Bzdusek K, Lock M and Chen J 2013 Automated IMRT planning with regional optimization using planning scripts *J. Appl. Clin. Med. Phys.* **14** 4052
[31] Wang H and Xing L 2016 Application programming in C# environment with recorded user software interactions and its application in autopilot of VMAT/IMRT treatment planning *J. Appl. Clin. Med. Phys.* **17** 189–203
[32] Hansen C R, Bertelsen A, Hazell I, Zukauskaite R, Gyldenkerne N and Johansen J *et al* 2016 Automatic treatment planning improves the clinical quality of head and neck cancer treatment plans *Clin. Transl. Radiat. Oncol.* **1** 2–8
[33] Hazell I, Bzdusek K, Kumar P, Hansen C R, Bertelsen A and Eriksen J G *et al* 2016 Automatic planning of head and neck treatment plans *J. Appl. Clin. Med. Phys.* **17** 272–82
[34] Xing L, Li J G, Pugachev A, Le Q T and Boyer A L 1999 Estimation theory and model parameter selection for therapeutic treatment plan optimization *Med. Phys.* **26** 2348–58
[35] Kalantzis G and Apte A 2014 A novel reduced-order prioritized optimization method for radiation therapy treatment planning *IEEE Trans. Biomed. Eng.* **61** 1062–70
[36] Clark V H, Chen Y, Wilkens J, Alaly J R, Zakaryan K and Deasy J O 2008 IMRT treatment planning for prostate cancer using prioritized prescription optimization and mean-tail-dose functions *Linear Algeb. Appl.* **428** 1345–64
[37] Wilkens J J, Alaly J R, Zakarian K, Thorstad W L and Deasy J O 2007 IMRT treatment planning based on prioritizing prescription goals *Phys. Med. Biol.* **52** 1675–92
[38] Breedveld S, Storchi P R M, Keijzer M, Heemink A W and Heijmen B J M 2007 A novel approach to multi-criteria inverse planning for IMRT *Phys. Med. Biol.* **52** 6339–53
[39] Jee K-W, McShan D L and Fraass B A 2007 Lexicographic ordering: intuitive multicriteria optimization for IMRT *Phys. Med. Biol.* **52** 1845–61
[40] Zarepisheh M, Hong L, Zhou Y, Oh J H, Mechalakos J G and Hunt M A *et al* 2019 Automated intensity modulated treatment planning: the expedited constrained hierarchical optimization (ECHO) system *Med. Phys.* **46** 2944–54
[41] Craft D L, Halabi T F, Shih H A and Bortfeld T R 2006 Approximating convex pareto surfaces in multiobjective radiotherapy planning *Med. Phys.* **33** 3399–407
[42] Craft D and Bortfeld T 2008 How many plans are needed in an IMRT multi-objective plan database? *Phys. Med. Biol.* **53** 2785–96

[43] Craft D L, Hong T S, Shih H A and Bortfeld T R 2012 Improved planning time and plan quality through multicriteria optimization for intensity-modulated radiotherapy *Int. J. Radiat. Oncol. Biol. Phys.* **82** e83–90

[44] Huang C, Yang Y, Panjwani N and Xing L 2021 Pareto Optimal Projection Search (POPS): automated radiation therapy treatment planning by direct search of the pareto surface *IEEE Trans. Biomed. Eng.* **68** 2907–17

[45] Huang C, Yang Y and Xing L 2021 Fully automated noncoplanar radiation therapy treatment planning arXiv: 2104.00784

[46] Nelder J A and Mead R 1965 A simplex method for function minimization *Comput. J.* **7** 308–13

[47] Huang C 2022 Developing automated tools in radiation therapy to streamline treatment planning and improve plan quality (Stanford, CA: Stanford University)

IOP Publishing

Artificial Intelligence in Radiation Therapy

Iori Sumida

Chapter 7

Artificial intelligence in adaptive radiation therapy

Yi Wang, Bin Cai, Leigh Conroy and X Sharon Qi

Adaptive radiation therapy (ART) is a personalized treatment using a feedback process to account for patient-specific anatomic, biological and/or functional changes during radiation therapy for cancer patients. ART can be implemented offline, online, or in real time, based on images acquired prior to or during the treatment. Once treatment adaptation is deemed necessary, the original treatment plan will be re-optimized (i.e., adapted) to deliver the optimal dosimetry to account for the changes. There are two major barriers for routine clinical implementation of ART: (1) the complexity of workflow and lack of efficient and robust tools; and (2) the limited available clinical resources such as staffing. Recently, the rapid advances of artificial intelligence (AI) technologies and the clinical applications of AI-assisted tools have significantly promoted the efficiency in every step of the ART workflow, accelerating the implementation of ART in many clinics. This chapter will focus on describing how AI technologies and AI-assisted tools can facilitate each step in the ART workflow, and reporting the latest technological advances of AI-ART. The basics of AI and its general applications on radiation therapy can be found in detail in other chapters.

7.1 Introduction

Adaptive radiation therapy (ART) is a closed-loop radiation treatment process where the initial treatment plan may be modified, via frequent imaging acquisition such as daily, using a systematic feedback of measurements [1–3]. It was first introduced to radiation oncology by Yan *et al* in 1997 [1]. Originally, ART is defined to improve radiation treatment by systematically monitoring treatment variations and incorporating them to re-optimize the treatment plan early on during the course of treatment. However, the definition of ART has evolved and broadened over the years. Currently, ART can be more formally defined as radiation therapy (RT) process where the delivered dose is systematically monitored during the course of treatment and modified as needed with the goal of improving clinical outcomes. With on-board 3D volumetric image guidance, ART allows assessment and modification of the original treatment plan to account for changes in target and orangs at risk (OARs), including both anatomical changes (e.g., size, shape, and patient weight), function and biology responses with the hope of minimizing normal tissue complication probability (NTCP) while maximizing tumor control probability (TCP) [4].

ART is now an established clinical practice in a number of treatment sites (e.g., head-and-neck, lung and abdomen). ART can be implemented offline, usually on a new simulation image, with decision on adaptation facilitated by systematical monitoring of anatomical and dosimetric variations. A more significant ART application is online, based on in-room volumetric images (e.g., CBCT or MRI) acquired immediately prior to the treatment delivery. ART can also be conducted in real time, while the treatment is being delivered, using real-time image tracking.

ART is expected to improve treatment quality by systematically monitoring treatment variations and incorporating them to re-optimize the treatment plan early on during the course of treatment. Despite these appealing advantages, clinical implementation of ART, especially online ART, has been limited due to its complexity and lack of efficient and robust software tools in almost every step of the process. The major barriers of preventing widespread of clinical implementation of ART in current practice can be briefly summarized as (1) the tedious and time-consuming workflow; (2) the limited clinical resources (i.e., staffing requirement); (3) the lack of a clinical decision support system [5]; and (4) the lack of comprehensive evidence on the clinical benefits (e.g., TCP, NTCP). Robust automation tools such as those assisted by AI are essential for routine clinical use of online ART without inducing treatment delay or excessive burden to staff.

The benefits of rapid advances of AI technologies and big data platforms have been harvested by a wide variety of medical disciplines, with pioneering work performed in pattern recognition and diagnosis assistance. The rapid developments of AI-assisted tools have demonstrated the values in terms of capability, flexibility, and efficiency in many clinical tasks in radiation oncology, and hold great promise in every aspects of ART workflow, including auto-segmentation of target and OARs, automated dose prediction and treatment planning, personalization of treatment based on quantitative imaging and genomics biomarkers, automatic clinical decision support, and automated quality control (QC) and quality assurance (QA). In addition, the operational efficiency gained by using AI-assisted tools in traditional, non-adaptive RT has freed up valuable clinical resources enabling wider adoption of online ART.

7.1.1 Advantages of ART

Image-guided radiation therapy (IGRT) has become the standard RT practice in many parts of the world, as it improves patient setup and enables accurate and precise delivery, leading to the widening of therapeutic radio [6, 7]. Standard IGRT practice generally consists of the following steps: (1) the acquisition of a volumetric treatment image prior to each treatment fraction, (2) registration of the treatment image with the planning image and (3) couch shift and rotation to accurately setup the target in a reproduceable position. In typical IGRT, the same initial RT plan is often delivered over the entire treatment course assuming inter-fractional/intra-fractional anatomical variations are minimal and can be corrected through couch movement. However, for some patients with certain diseases, couch movement alone may not be enough to account for the changes in the size or shape of the tumor volume and/or OARs, or overall patient weight gain or loss. Such changes, identifiable on daily treatment image, forces clinicians to use large uncertainty margin (e.g., 5 mm to 10 mm) and low fractional dose (typically, 1.8 Gy to 2 Gy) to assure the safety and limit normal organ toxicity. Other than anatomical variations, functional changes based on daily images, especially with the emergence of in-room MR and PET imaging [8, 9], pose the next layer of clinical needs for ART.

ART can maximize the therapeutic ratio by further increasing tumor dose while maintaining or even reducing normal tissue complication. Early studies on ART have already provided promising evidence on enabling dose escalation, reduced toxicity and potential improvement of clinical outcomes across multiple disease sites [10–13]. Chen *et al* [10] studied the effect of adaptive re-planning on clinical outcomes for 317 head-and-neck patients, who underwent IMRT with daily IGRT for newly diagnosed squamous cell carcinoma to a median dose of 66 Gy (ranging from 60 Gy to74 Gy). Among these patients, 51 (16%) underwent ART with one plan modification midway through the treatment. This study suggested a significant benefit in appropriately selected patients for ART, while the use of routine re-planning is probably not necessary. To facilitate adaptive decision making for H&N RT, Qi *et al* [5] developed a near real-time framework allowing for systematic assessment of anatomic variations and dosimetric variations using a GPU-based dose deformation framework to improve treatment efficacy, which enables timely plan adaptation leading to potential outcome improvement.

7.1.2 Types of ART, current status and challenges

Depending on the re-planning scenarios and time scales, there are three general types of ART [4]: offline, online, and real-time ART. The offline ART indicates that the re-planning process occurs offline and between fractions. The original treatment might be continued while the team members carry out the re-planning process. The adapted plan will be scheduled for the next available fraction. The possible large inter-fraction changes pose a big challenge for offline ART. The re-planning effort might be diminished due to large day-to-day variations. The online ART typically occurs right before treatment while contours are re-drawn based on the daily image and the plan is re-optimized to meet clinical goals. The patient remains on the table during the re-planning progresses and the adapted plan will be delivered immediately upon completion of the adaptive re-planning workflow. The challenges for online ART are the possible intra-fraction changes due to organ filings and motions. The real-time adaptive planning occurs during a fraction, where the monitoring of anatomical changes and correction on doses happens simultaneously during radiation delivery [14]. The plan is essentially adapted in real time with a modified dose delivered to the patient in response to target or organ changes. The real-time ART is the ultimate form of ART enabling more accurate tumor targeting and OARs sparing but relies heavily on technology for reliable target tracking, rapid re-planning and robust quality assurance (QA). The offline ART has been already used by many clinics when clinically significant changes are observed in treatment course. For online ART, several CT or MR guided RT platforms are commercially available and have been implemented by early adopters [15–17]. Currently, there is no clinically available commercial system designed for real-time ART, and the robust real-time tracking and dose shaping remain as popular developmental topics for many research groups.

7.1.3 Overview of current workflow of ART and current challenges

As shown in figure 7.1, there are five major steps in the online and offline ART workflow: (1) imaging acquisition and segmentation, (2) dose assessment and adaptation decision making, (3) plan re-optimization, (4) quality control (QC) and quality assurance (QA), and (5) plan delivery.

High-quality imaging systems that can detect the changes of target and OARs are the foundations of ART. Currently, CT or MR systems remain the major imaging modalities used in ART. Biological imaging, such as PET, also has promising applications for some disease sites. The daily images for ART need to have minimal artifacts and good integrity from a physics point of view, as well as be easy to contour for clinicians. Besides imaging quality, rapid image acquisition is also desired for online and real-time ART. The assessment step includes evaluation of structure changes and possible re-contouring. Depending on the treatment site and daily changes, after assessment, a portion or all the structures need to be re-contoured. Currently, this is the most time-consuming step in ART due to lack of automation. The re-planning step occurs right after the contours are confirmed. The flexibility of re-planning depends on the type of ART. A total re-plan (different beam arrangement, delivery technique and constraints) is possible for offline ART. However, limited options are available for online and real-time ART. Usually only re-optimization and/or re-adjustment of beam aperture is performed. The delivery part is very similar to the standard IGRT for offline and online ART, but is different for real-time ART. Reliable imaging tracking, fast re-assessment and quick adjustment during the delivery process is critical for real-time ART. It is worth mentioning that, within each step of ART, the appropriate QA/QC measures are also required to ensure a safe and high-quality delivery of ART.

Clinical implementation of ART involves systematical monitoring and analyzing of daily images. ART is generally labor-intensive and time-consuming, leading to

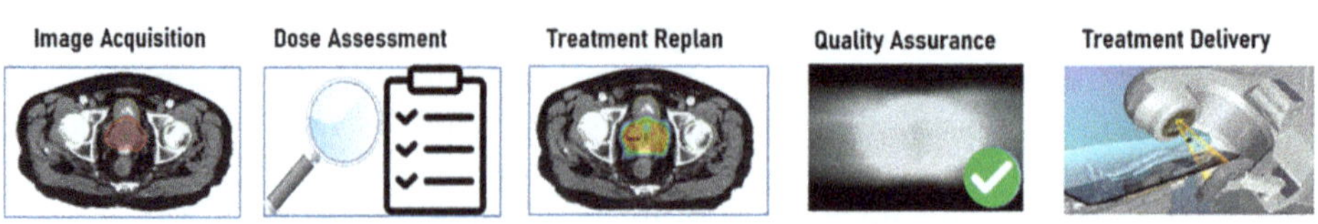

Figure 7.1. Typical ART workflow with five major steps.

additional risks to standard IGRT. From offline, to online, to real time ART, the complexity of workflow and requirement on technologies increases dramatically. To safely complete all steps of ART within a short timescale is the biggest challenge. The rapid advances of AI technologies have demonstrated that it can increase capability, flexibility, and efficiency in many clinical tasks in RT [18, 19].

7.1.4 AI and AI-assisted technologies for ART

AI uses complex computer algorithms to mimic human capabilities and create human-like intelligence, including visual perception, pattern recognition, decision-making, and problem solving. AI can help humans solve complex problems and promote efficiency via automation. AI is currently emerging in many fields of medicine and healthcare. The emerging opportunities offered by AI have been widely recognized by both academia and industry. While the RT industry is providing more and more diversified AI-driven platforms to assist every step in the RT workflow, researchers from academia are building more AI models to mimic the clinical expertise. The rapid integration of AI in the traditional RT workflow is not only improving the quality, efficiency and safety of the treatment, but also freeing up valuable clinical resources for ART implementation.

ART is a premium target for using AI in radiation oncology. While many venders are providing AI solutions for almost every step in the traditional RT workflow (e.g., auto-segmentation, auto-planning, plan checking), some tools are also being adapted and upgraded to facilitate ART.

Online ART has a unique character. It requires a substantial amount of work in a very short time. AI not only plays an important role to automate the ART workflow, but also promotes consistency and objectivity in clinical decision making. For example, the AI-driven auto-image registration includes no observer bias and the automated calculations of region of interest (ROI) volume and dose changes trigger pre-defined thresholds when clinically significant deviation occurs. In addition, analyzing inter-fraction changes from daily IGRT images is currently done by a human observer from the ART team (e.g., radiation therapist, medical physicist, or physician) in a very subjective and qualitative manner, which is also labor-intensive. The observer determines the need for ART simply by visually inspecting the IGRT image and grossly identifying macroscopic anatomic changes relative to the original planning image, often without rigorously evaluating the dosimetric impact. AI-assisted tools can analyze the inter-fraction changes and automatically evaluate the resulting dosimetric impact, and thus help to determine the need for ART in an objective and quantitative manner. In addition to improved quality and efficiency, AI can also be used to optimize the quality assurance (QA) and quality control (QC) processes to promote the safety of online ART.

7.2 The role of AI in ART workflow

AI is playing an increasing and more important role in every step of the ART workflow. As previously described, in offline ART, a new simulation image is often acquired, and a new treatment plan is generated in a similar manner to initial planning. Therefore, the applications of AI for offline ART are very similar to that for initial planning, and thus the reader can refer to other chapters for more details. This section will focus on explaining the AI applications for online ART. The real-time ART is of great developmental interest, but some time away from routine clinical adoption.

Figure 7.2 provides a closer look at the online ART workflow. The steps in the red box are expanded from the general workflow shown in figure 7.1. These steps are done with the patient on the couch. The post-delivery dose evaluation and correction, done offline after the treatment, are unique to online ART, as the current online adaptive plan needs to be taken into account in the next adaptive fraction [17].

AI technologies have been used to facilitate each step in the online ART workflow. (1) The online ART starts with taking daily images using in-room CBCT or MRI. Deep neural network can be used to improve the image quality of CBCT by reducing scatter. Once the daily image is acquired, machine learning algorithms can be used to generate pseudo-CT images from CBCT or MRI to provide more accurate information on electron density and allow a CT-based auto-segmentation model to be used directly. (2) As the most advanced tool for auto-segmentation, deep learning is also powerful at propagating initial contours onto daily images via deformable image registration or re-contouring all ROIs given the knowledge of the initial contours. (3) While daily adaptation can help prevent significant dose deviation, it is also subject to addition uncertainties on segmentation and optimization resulting from the inferior quality of the in-room images, compared to the high-quality simulation CT or MRI images. Therefore, it is important for a machine learning-based decision support system to assess the dosimetric impact on daily adaptation. (4) If daily adaptation is warranted, AI-based auto-planning tools (e.g., knowledge-based planning from Varian, machine learning optimization from RaySearch) can quickly re-optimize the pre-plan (which could be the initial treatment plan, the latest offline adaptive plan, or the last online adaptive plan) to account for the daily anatomical, functional or biological

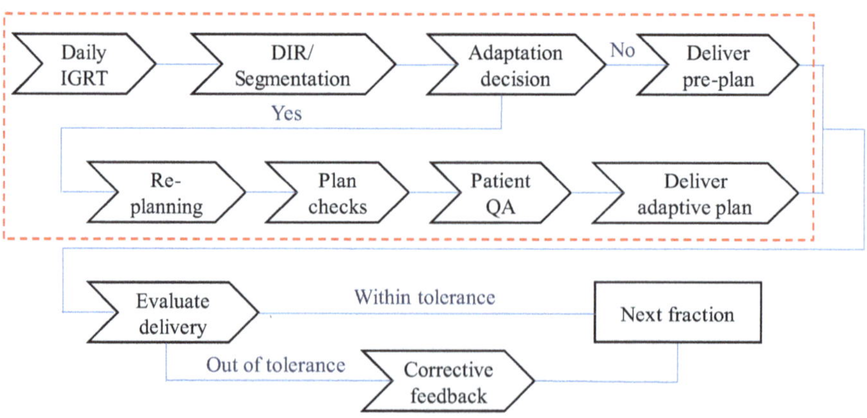

Figure 7.2. Example of online ART workflow.

variation. (5) While the patient is on the couch, machine learning-based solutions on plan quality control, secondary verification, and AI-based plan error detection and plan check tools can help speed up this process. (6) Prior to the initial delivery, regulation requires quality assurance (QA) measurement of the patient plan. As such measurement is difficult with the patient on the couch, machine learning models can be built to predict the passing rate, given the knowledge of historical data, results of initial QA, character of the daily plan and daily performance of the treatment machine (e.g., MLC position). (7) After delivery, the delivered plan needs to be evaluated and the dose should be accumulated for future fractions. If any dosimetry is out of tolerance, corrective feedback needs to be provided for future fractions, if there is any fraction left.

7.2.1 Deep learning for improving in-room image quality and generating pseudo-CT

Online ART is based on in-room imaging modalities, most often, CBCT or MRI. The quality of the online adaptation is limited by the quality of the in-room image. The quality of the CBCT image is inferior to the original planning CT, mainly due to increase scatter radiation. The quality of the in-room MRI image is limited by the strength of the magnetic field, which is often 3 T for an MRI simulator and up to 1.5 T for the in-room MRI. While it could be possible to increase the magnetic field strength to 3 T for in-room MRI to match the simulator, it is unlikely that in-room CT (which was previously investigated) will gain much popularity. The quality of the CBCT image can be improved by placing a metal anti-scatter collimator above the detector, or via algorithms that correct scatter on each projection image or the reconstructed image. Many scatter correction strategies have been investigated for CBCT, among which the deep learning methods have shown great potential in learning complex relationships and incorporating existing knowledge into the model through feature extraction and representation learning. When trained by many paired projection and scatter images, a deep learning model can produce a powerful non-linear prediction of scatter distribution. Maier *et al* proposed a convolutional neural network (CNN, a class of deep neural network commonly used to analyze visual imagery)-based scatter correction for industrial CBCT applications [18]. Hansen *et al* demonstrated that CNN-based CBCT intensity correction improved photon dose distribution calculation accuracy [19]. Nomura *et al* developed an effective scatter correction method using a residual CNN [20]. Podgorsak *et al* used generative adversarial networks (GAN, in which two models are trained simultaneously: a generative model *G* capturing data distribution and a discriminative model *D* estimating the probability that a sample came from the training data rather than *G*) to correct for CBCT artifact arising from sparse and truncated projection data [21].

Traditionally, treatment planning is done on a simulation CT image, which provides the most accurate electron density information. In addition, most current auto-segmentation and auto-planning models, which are critical components for fast treatment adaptation, were developed on CT images. Therefore, many researchers have investigated the generation of pseudo-CT images from CBCT or in-room MRI.

On the CBCT side, Liang *et al* developed a cycle-consistent generative adversarial network framework (Cycle-GAN, a technique involving automatic training of image-to-image translation models without paired examples) to synthesize CT images from CBCT images [22]. This model is capable of image-to-image translation using unpaired CT and CBCT images in an unsupervised learning setting. The synthetic CT images generated from CBCT through this Cycle-GAN model are visually and quantitatively similar to real CT. Chen *et al* used a deep U-net-based approach to synthesize CT-like images with accurate numbers from planning CT, while keeping the same anatomical structure as on-treatment CBCT [23]. Harms *et al* integrated a residual block concept into a cycle-GAN framework, called res-cycle-GAN, to learn a mapping between CBCT images and paired planning CT images [24]. Compared with a GAN, a cycle-GAN includes an inverse transformation from CBCT to CT images, which constrains the model by forcing calculation of both a CBCT and a synthetic CBCT.

On the MRI side, a variety of methods (e.g., patch-based, atlas-based and bulk density assignment) have been investigated for pseudo-CT generation. Two methods have been clinically implemented. One directly uses deformable image registration (DIR) to a pre-treatment CT, while the other uses bulk assignment in combination with DIR [25].

7.2.2 Deep learning for deformable image registration and auto-segmentation

Deep learning has been widely investigated for auto-segmentation and commercialized by several leading RT vendors (e.g., Mirada, RaySearch, and Varian). Most RT auto-segmentation solutions utilize a U-Net architecture (named after its u-shape structure), which consists of a contracting path (regular CNN providing image classification) and an expansion path (up-convolutions and concatenations with features from the contracting path). These solutions have provided comparable or even preferable auto-contours over manually drawn contours for OARs for several disease sites (e.g., head-and-neck, thorax and prostate). For ART, it usually requires the target(s) and ROIs on new images to be segmented, such as a new CT simulation for offline ART, or CBCTs and daily MRIs for online ART, reflecting patient's anatomical changes to ensure accurate dose calculation and dose accumulation during the course of treatment delivery. Accurate and efficient segmentation is generally crucial as they were generally used to assess dose delivery and/or re-optimize in an ART workflow. auto-segmentation on CBCT has also been widely investigated. Varian has demonstrated substantial improvement on CBCT image quality on its most advanced AI-driven ART platform—the Ethos system. Sibolt *et al* from one of Varian first Ethos testing sites reported their clinical experience on using the Ethos system for online ART in the pelvic region [26]. The AI-driven influencer segmentation required approximately 3–6 min and a review of propagated CTVs was carried out within an additional 1–3 min Elmahdy developed a robust contour propagation using deep learning and image registration and tested it for online adaptive proton therapy of prostate cancer [27].

7.2.3 Machine learning for decision support on daily adaptation

After getting contours of tumor volumes and OARs on the daily image, the ART team faces a decision on whether to deliver the pre-treatment plan (initial plan, last offline adaptive plan, or the adaptive plan from the last fraction) or the adaptive plan of the day. On the one hand, re-optimization based on the daily image is in theory always beneficial compared to using the pre-plan, considering anatomical, functional and biological variations, organ motion and setup error. However, on the other hand, the benefit starts to decline with more interval between the time of imaging and the time of the delivery. Moreover, the segmentation and fast re-planning on the daily image are always subject to more uncertainties, due to the inferior quality of the daily image. Therefore, it is essential to have a quantified system to aid the clinical decision on treatment adaptation. While simple geometric threshold is useful to make a quick decision, more comprehensive information on dosimetry and clinical outcome can bring the benefits of treatment adaptation to a higher level and provide more concrete justification on the use of the more expensive online ART approach.

Guidi *et al* developed an expert system classifier to identify the situations in need of re-planning intervention in online ART, based on daily anatomical and dosimetric variations [28]. The model learned from historical data and can mimic past practice. It cannot determine the benefit based on treatment outcome. El Naqa *et al* used reinforcement learning to build a knowledge-based decision-making model for ART [20, 21] and tested it on patients with liver and lung cancers. The model was first flexibly trained to learn representations of the radiotherapy state space, and then optimize treatment outcome based on diagnostic, dosimetric, biological, and genetic features and using reward functions incorporating clinical protocols and prior clinical knowledge. The model's decision was comparable to those made by clinicians.

7.2.4 Machine learning for online re-optimization

Adaptive re-planning is the central piece of online treatment adaptation. It requires fast optimization to tune the latest treatment plan, either from initial planning or offline adaptation, to optimize the treatment of the day. While the initial or offline plans are often done with inverse optimization, a fresh start is neither needed nor preferred for online adaptation with patient on the couch. In the online ART setting, machine leaning auto-planning models can learn from historical treatments and their adaptations and apply the tuning to the daily volumes. The model also needs to consider all prior fractions and optimize the overall treatment up to the day of treatment.

Varian's AI-driven ART system, Ethos, can automatically re-optimize the treatment plan to the daily contours. Varian also has the AI-driven auto-planning solution—knowledge-based planning (KPB), which predicts the dose-volume histogram (DVH) of different structures based on their geometric relationship to the target.

RaySearch offers a machine learning optimization (MLO) framework, first based on a random forest algorithm, and later a deep neural network. The MLO algorithm can predict 3D voxel dose distribution, mimic the distribution to generate a directly deliverable auto-plan. In RayStation 10B, an MLO plan is generated in six iterations. The first five iterations can be saved as the starting point for fast online re-optimization, assuming the daily anatomy will not be significantly different from that in the pre-treatment plan.

7.2.5 AI for quality assurance, verification, and error detection

QA, verification, and error detection in the traditional RT treatment workflow is often a highly manual and time-consuming process. In online ART, workflows are expediated and there is increased time pressure; as a result, there is a need for integrated AI-enhanced QA and error detection to ensure the safe and timely delivery of adapted treatments. Mixed-methods of error detection (e.g., manual, rules-based automation, AI-based) may best support the clinical ART workflow. For example, basic data comparison tasks will benefit more from rule-based automation, whereas complex decision making, and context-specific checks performed by a human may be augmented by AI for increased efficacy.

A challenge in AI-based error detection in radiotherapy is the class-imbalance between erroneous and non-erroneous data. Clinically, once an error is identified, it is immediately corrected, and there is no capture of the error-containing data for algorithm training. The creation of false errors for training may introduce biases not reflected in the real-world data. As a result, many QA and error-detection algorithms focus on outlier detection. Ideally, error detection and QA algorithms intended for use with ART will be trained using historical data from the workflow; however, large ART datasets may not be available. Active curation of adaptive cases with real-world errors is useful for QA algorithm validation and testing. AI-algorithms for QA should be tested for continued relevance and ability to detect errors. Furthermore, algorithms require periodic updates to avoid flagging intentional changes in practice as errors [22]. Finally, if aspects of the adaptation are generated by an AI algorithm, the algorithm used for QA should be completely independent in method and training data [23].

Online adaptive workflows are performed while the patient is in the treatment position, resulting in condensed timelines compared to traditional QA. QA algorithms should be fast, relevant to the clinical context, and seamlessly integrated. Presented information about flagged errors or suboptimality provided by a QA algorithm must be timely, relevant, and actionable for decision making. End users should be trained to interpret algorithm outputs and should understand the capabilities and limitations of the AI.

7.2.6 AI for physics plan check

In traditional RT workflows, physics plan check has been demonstrated to be one of the most valuable QA steps [24]. The purpose of physics plan QA is to evaluate the acceptability of the RT treatment plan against the clinical context and treatment intent, investigate deviations from clinical norms and protocols, detect errors in treatment planning, and to assess the deliverability of the plan. Physics plan check is a comprehensive evaluation of all preceding work, including image quality, registration accuracy, contour acceptability, treatment plan optimization, plan delivery, and data transfer. Traditionally, this QA step occurs at the end of the treatment planning process, with minimal involvement from physics in the upstream steps. In offline adaptive workflows this conventional plan check workflow can be applied with minimal alteration. In online ART, manual physics QA after completion of all planning steps is too laborious for practical use. Time savings can be realized by integrating QA and error detection within the process, so that errors can be detected and corrected immediately, and re-work is minimized.

Simple rule-based plan check items, such as data transfer, can be easily automated without machine learning algorithms. However, rule-based automation approaches do not handle outlying cases well as each potential outlier case requires hardcoding into the algorithm. Conversely, many aspects of physics plan check require specific clinical expertise and expert judgment to assesses the quality and appropriateness of the plan with respect to the individual patient context and institutional standards of practice. AI can be used to expediate, assist, and augment this human evaluation.

Contours are among the highest-risk errors that can be detected during physics plan QA [25] because they are used both to drive optimization and in plan evaluation. Automated segmentation of organs-at-risk (OARs) in online ART may be based on the registration of the reference planning and daily adaptive images. The contours must then be manually verified and modified. AI-based automated contouring offers significant time savings in online ART; however, the output of such automation often requires manual editing and increased scrutiny. Manual contour review can be time-consuming and labor-intensive, requiring slice-by-slice review of each contour. The contour review process is also prone to error due to possible inattention or lack of experience. Automated contour QA may expediate and improve ART workflows. Registration-based propagation and automated contouring algorithms can produce contouring errors that are fundamentally different from those that would happen with human delineation [26]; therefore, any AI for contour QA must be trained to detect errors using contours generated according to the clinical ART process [27]. Furthermore, if OARs are auto-segmented using AI-based automated contouring, the algorithm used to evaluate the contours should be completely independent in function and training data from the algorithm used to generate the contours [23].

Common contouring errors include mislabeling, missed slices, isolated voxels and large area changes between slices. With human-generated contours, the high inter- and intra-contouring variation within contours without errors makes automated contour error detection a difficult task. McIntosh *et al* [28] demonstrated a random forest classification technique to flag mislabeled or erroneous contours. The algorithm used sets of decision trees to learn the probability of a region of interest (ROI) belonging to a class of ROIs given its feature set consisting of shape and density features calculated for each ROI individually and between ROIs. Chen *et al* [29] developed an automatic contour error-detection strategy based on inter- and intra-structural geometric attribute distribution (GAD) models for head-and-neck contours. Based on ROI-specific features and relationships between neighboring ROIs, principal component analysis (PCA) was used to determine the geometric attribute spaces based on samples of correct contours and the resultant model was used to detect outliers. As part of this error-detection algorithm, Chen *et al* developed an interactive visual interface to aid with identification and correction of the detected errors. AI output interpretability for fast detection and correction of flagged contours will be critical for QA in adaptive workflows where time to search for the source of the failed QA result is limited. An alternate approach to AI-based contour QA for automatically generated contours is to integrate a measure of confidence into the auto-segmentation algorithm to flag for manual review or edits [30]. Finally, Rhee *et al* [26] developed a convolutional neural network (CNN) automated contouring approach to flag suspicious contours generated by their multi-atlas-based auto-contouring system (MACS), classifying detected contouring errors as either minor or major. The two auto-contouring algorithms (generation MACS and verification CNN) were completely independent.

The increasing complexity of and number of variables within modern RT planning makes manual treatment plan QA challenging. In online ART, a physicist may be physically present during re-planning, which can decrease the workload of the end-of-planning physics check. Additionally, the newly generated plan of the day is often based on a reference plan with similar features (e.g., isocenter, beam angles, etc), which can further reduce the daily plan QA burden. Radiation treatment plans are highly individualized to the patient, and as a result physics plan QA can be subjective and dependent upon available time and expertise. One of the most challenging aspects of physics plan QA is determining if the plan is as good as it could be with the respect to the individual patient anatomy. This challenge is further compounded in ART, where iterative alteration of the optimization parameters may consume valuable time while the patient is on the treatment couch. To realize the full clinical potential of ART, the daily adapted plan should be of equivalent quality as traditional plans despite the expediated workflow. AI-based QA tools have the potential to augment the physics plan check by flagging plans with differences from historical data for human review for reduced QA burden and improved error-detection rate.

Azmandian *et al* [31], used a K-means clustering algorithm to cluster simple historical plans based on a small number of treatment parameters (beam energy and monitor units) and demonstrated the feasibility of detecting large errors in RT plans using this approach. The algorithm was completely independent of the treatment planning system and highlighted the outlying parameter to aid with error correction. Modern ART plans are more complicated, with many more variables, than the four-field-box plans that were evaluated in this study. Luk *et al* [22], has demonstrated the use of a Bayesian network (BN) to flag outlying plans based on a larger number of plan variables. The BN is a network of jointly dependent plan parameters that mimics human reasoning in determining plan appropriateness for a given patient by assessing the probability of the set of plan parameters given the diagnostic information, based on what has been learned from the historical training set [32].

For a new input plan, the network can identify unusual or error-containing plan parameters and flag those parameters for manual review. A BN for online ART would be likely to need to be specifically constructed or learned from ART data, since data, parameter relationships and error modes may differ from traditional practice.

Knowledge-based dose prediction has shown promise for automated QA of the dosimetric appropriateness of a plan for a novel patient [33–35]. Knowledge-based dose prediction provides a statistical range of acceptable dose-volume statistics for a novel input patient based on relationships between ROI geometry features and dose statistics learned from previously-delivered treatment plans. In adaptive planning, patient anatomy could be more or less favorable than that of the reference plan on a given day. Knowledge-based dose prediction could be used to guide online planning objectives and evaluate the appropriateness of the plan to identify when further manual tuning would be beneficial based on the daily anatomy. Training data for knowledge-based models should be carefully curated to ensure high-quality planning recommendations.

In any AI-based plan QA algorithm applied to ART, the aim of the algorithm will be to augment the human plan review by flagging plan discrepancies based on historical data for manual review. The output of the algorithm should be easily interpretable and immediately actionable. Those using the algorithm outputs must be educated in what types of errors the algorithm can and cannot detect, and the limitation of the AI.

7.2.7 Considerations for education and training

As with any new process or technology, staff education and training for AI-enabled workflows is paramount for successful clinical translation and execution. The introduction of AI into radiotherapy workflows is not unique to ART; however, the short timelines and multidisciplinary nature of online ART workflows emphasizes the importance of training and education of those who will be making clinical decisions based on outputs from an AI system. The introduction of AI into an ART workflow will automate and remove tasks; however, a new required competence emerges: all clinical users should have knowledge of how to correctly use the AI and should understand the limitations and pitfalls [36]. A multidisciplinary competency-based training program should be developed to ensure that the ART team knows the required inputs, understands limitations, and can identify erroneous outputs [36–38]. AI-enabled ART processes should have integrated quality assurance of the AI outputs with a corresponding workflow design dictating clear actions to be taken if the AI fails or produces erroneous results.

7.3 Existing AI solutions for ART

In this section, several currently available integrated AI solutions designed for ART are introduced and reviewed, including ETHOS treatment planning and delivery system (Varian Medical System, Palo Alto, CA), RayStation treatment planning system (RaySearch Laboratories, Stockholm, Sweden), as well as Accuray PreciseART (Accuray Inc., Sunnyvale, CA) software.

7.3.1 Ethos online ART platform from Varian medical

Ethos™ treatment platform is the latest integrated ART solution developed by Varian Medical System (Palo Alto, CA). One of the design goals for the Ethos system is to provide a rapid and robust CBCT-guided online ART which can be delivered in 15 min to 30 min Ethos therapy comprises three fully integrated components: Ethos radiotherapy system, Ethos treatment management, and Ethos treatment planning system. The foundation of Ethos therapy is the adaptive intelligence, which utilizes AI tools to facilitate the ART process and to achieve a more precise treatment. As shown in figure 7.3, on the hardware side, it is coupled with a compact medical linear accelerator (linac) with a rapid rotation ring gantry. The machine can provide 6 MV flattering-filter-free photon beam. Other innovative technologies include a cutting-edge double-stack multi-leaf collimator (MLC), a high-quality kilo-voltage (kV) CBCT system and a robust workflow to deliver highly efficient and precise radiotherapy treatment. On the software side, Ethos utilizes an integrated treatment planning and monitoring system (TPMS) with AI tools to help organ contours, plan optimization, and treatment monitoring.

The adaptive treatment started with acquisition of high-quality kV CBCT images. There are 11 preset imaging protocols with the fastest images acquired in 17 s. After image acquisition, the system automatically segments the OARs and generates the target volumes. After all contours of organs and targets are confirmed by clinicians or adapters, the system automatically generates two plans: scheduled plan and adaptive plan. The scheduled plan is the initial plan calculated based on anatomy from the image of the day, whereas the adapted plan is the original plan re-optimized based on the preset clinical constraints. In the plan review workspace, the users can easily assess the plans based on preset plan metrics, dose distribution and DVH for each structure. While the plans are being reviewed, the system automatically send both plans to Mobius3D for a secondary dose calculation-based plan QA.

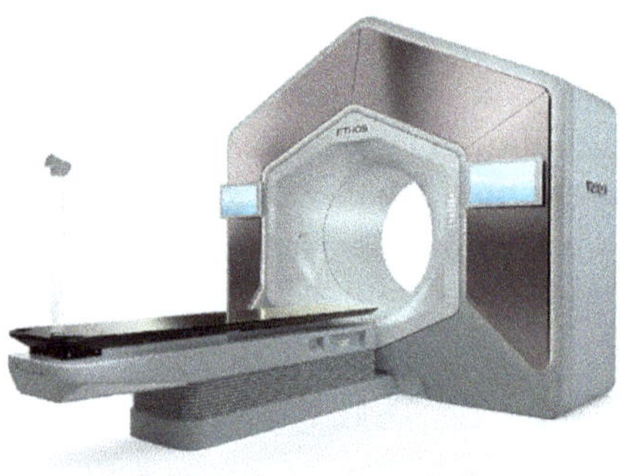

Figure 7.3. The Ethos™ ring gantry treatment machine. (Image courtesy of Varian Medical Systems, Inc., Palo Alto, CA. Copyright 2021. All rights reserved.)

The user will decide between scheduled plan and adaptive plan based on the dose distribution and constraints for treatment delivery.

Overall, on Ethos platform, the AI tools are primarily used for (1) auto-segmentation and (2) plan re-optimization.

The AI segmentation models were built based on a CNN with a training dataset provided by multiple institutes, and thoroughly validated by the vendor before clinical release. Ethos uses full image deep convolutional neural networks with proprietary architectures that share many similarities with U-Net and DenseNet (CNN with dense connections) [39–41]. The network itself takes the full 3D image dataset as input and returns the same size of segmentation as an output. Figure 7.4 shows the user interface of AI auto-segmentations during the online adaptation process. The clinicians have the opportunity to modify and conform the auto-segmentations done by AI before proceeding to the next step. In the current version, not all OARs have its corresponding AI modes and the availability of AI models depend on the disease site.

Some initial assessment work on Ethos AI auto-segmentation modes has been done by early adopters. For example, *Cai et al* [42] evaluated the efficiency and accuracy of AI auto-delineation via a prospective *in silico* CBCT-guided stereotactic online adaptive radiotherapy (CT-STAR) trial targeting upper abdominal malignancies. They simulated 23 fractions online adaptive treatment for five patients with 61 AI contours (23 liver, 15 stomach and 23 duodenum) generated and compared to the ground truth (physician manual contours). The average time required to complete the AI auto-contours of all three organs are 46.8±15 s. The auto-contours generated by AI only required minor or no editing 65% of the time for liver, 17% for stomach and 8.7% for duodenum. The post analysis indicated the mean Dice similarity coefficients (DSC) was 0.93±0.06 (median 0.94), 0.80±0.13 (median 0.85),

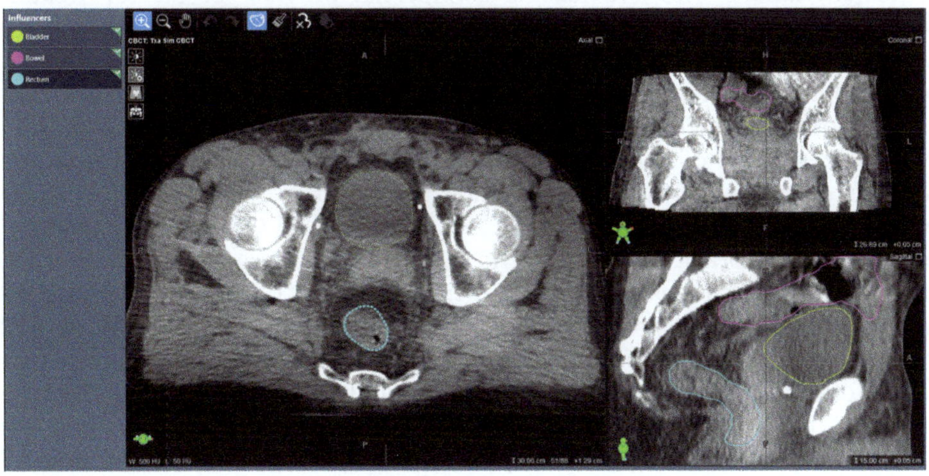

Figure 7.4. Ethos auto-segmentation interface for online adaptation. For this treatment, the bladder, bowel and rectum are auto-contoured by AI-assisted auto-segmentation tools which requires the clinician's confirmation before proceeding to target generation.

0.70 ± 0.18 (median 0.74) for liver, stomach and duodenum, respectively. The average distance between the AI and the ground truth manual contours are 1.42±1.56 mm (median 0.71 mm), 2.53 ± 1.54 mm (median 2.08 mm) and 3.52±1.97 mm (median 3.43 mm) for liver, stomach, and duodenum, respectively. These results indicated that the AI contours have high efficiency and the potential to facilitate online contouring for ART. Currently, the contouring accuracy is organ-dependent. For upper GI treatment site, the current AI models are more accurate for liver and stomach, but suboptimal for duodenum. This implies that a thorough verification by the clinical team is critical.

AI is also used to drive an intelligent optimizer engine (IOE). The IOE is used to drive the optimization process to achieve a list of preset clinical goals. The IOE first translates the clinical goals to objective functions and creates quality functions (Q-functions) to monitor the progress of optimization. For the optimization monitoring, the IOE iteratively works on the objective functions by pre-defined priority of each structure. Unfulfilled goals with higher priority receive attention before those of lower priority. When all goals are met, additional effort is to reduce the dose to OARs as much as possible. The ultimate goal of the IOE is to automatically generate an optimal plan meeting all clinical goals as quick as possible for online re-optimization.

Since it was released in 2019, the Ethos online adaptation platform has been adopted by institutes across the world. The AI components are among the core features to ensure a safe and high-quality delivery of ART on this platform. More validation works are in progress and clinical trials have also been proposed based on this system.

7.3.2 Machine learning solutions from RaySearch Laboratories

RaySearch Laboratories is a leading commercial provider of the RT treatment planning system and record and verification system. It has introduced comprehensive machine learning solutions for auto-segmentation and auto-planning for conventional, non-adaptive radiation therapy. Its development team has reported a deep learning algorithm with a GAN architecture to generate synthetic CT to allow the expansion of its existing machine learning solutions into the territory of ART. Its deep learning auto-segmentation algorithm uses a convolutional neural network with a U-Net architecture. So far it has released CT and MRI models for head-and-neck, thoracic and male pelvic treatment. Auto-segmentation takes about a minute. RaySearch was the first commercial provider of machine learning auto-planning solutions, first with a random forest algorithm in version 8B, and later upgraded to a deep neural network in version 10B. Machine learning auto-planning models for head-and-neck, thoracic, abdominal and pelvic treatment sites have been reported for photon and proton planning. These auto-segmentation and auto-planning models can be readily adapted to the ART applications. In non-ART auto-planning, the deep learning algorithm runs six iterations, with the last one focusing on fine adjustments to challenging goals. In ART application, the first five iterations can be saved and the six repeated for each online adaption.

7.3.3 PreciseART offline dose monitoring platform from Accuray

A commercially available package, PreciseART (Accuray Inc., Sunnyvale, CA) is an integrated MIM viewer (MIM Software, Inc., Cleveland, Ohio) especially designed for offline ART analyses, including dose monitoring, re-planning and delivery verification. It is a fully integrated and automated dose monitoring platform to streamline offline ART analyses and to create revised treatment plans on tomotherapy [43]. The package takes the following objects, including the plan CT, the planning structure set, the plan delivery beam intensity pattern (sinogram), daily megavoltage (MV) CT treatment images and daily patient registrations, as inputs. The daily dose is calculated upon each MVCT using the sinogram and the CT-number table associated with the MVCT scan at the time of treatment. A merged daily image is created using the planning CT to fill in the missing information in the superior, inferior, and axial portions not included in the daily MVCT.

After the patients enrolled into the offline ART program, there is no other user intervention required. Specifically, as soon as each fraction delivery is completed, the system automatically creates a merged daily image, deforms the plan ROI contours onto the daily image, calculates the dose on the daily image, accumulates the daily dose onto the plan CT, and generates a report with user-defined metrics, flags, and trends. The entire process takes approximately 15–20 min per fraction, depending on the size and resolution of the MVCT, making the report available shortly after the fraction delivery. Besides the daily dose that is calculated based on a single fraction MVCT, the accumulated dose (the accumulation of all prior fraction MVCT-recalculated doses), and the projected dose (the accumulated dose except it accumulates the dose up to the latest fraction and repeats the latest fraction for the remaining treatment course), are calculated and available for offline clinical decision making.

7.4 Summary

ART is a form of personalized treatment by systematically monitoring treatment variations and incorporating them to re-optimize the treatment plan early on during the course of treatment. A new paradigm of developing advanced AI technologies and AI-assisted automation shows great promise in each aspect of the ART workflow, including automated segmentation of the target and OARs, development of biomarkers for AI-ART; automated ART decision making frameworks built from deep learning neural networks, automated dose prediction and re-optimization, as well as the subsequent QC and QA processes. As the efficiency and effectiveness of AI and AI-assisted technologies continues to evolve, it is highly expected that the widespread clinical implementation of ART will lead to further improvement of clinical outcome.

References

[1] Yan D, Vicini F, Wong J and Martinez A 1997 Adaptive radiation therapy *Phys. Med. Biol.* **42** 123–32

[2] Yan D 2010 Adaptive radiotherapy: merging principle into clinical practice *Semin. Radiat. Oncol.* **20** 79–83

[3] Mutic S 2017 Automatic image segmentation and structure evaluation for on-line adaptive RT *Radiother. Oncol.* **123** S107–07

[4] Green O L, Henke L E and Hugo G D 2019 Practical clinical workflows for online and offline adaptive radiation therapy *Semin. Radiat. Oncol.* **20** 219–27

[5] Qi X S *et al* 2015 Near real-time assessment of anatomic and dosimetric variations for head and neck radiation therapy via graphics processing unit-based dose deformation framework *Int. J. Radiat. Oncol. Biol. Phys.* **92** 415–22

[6] Zelefsky M J, Kollmeier M, Cox B, Fidaleo A, Sperling D, Pei X, Carver B, Coleman J, Lovelock M and Hunt M 2012 Improved clinical outcomes with high-dose image guided radiotherapy compared with non-IGRT for the treatment of clinically localized prostate cancer *Int. J. Radiat. Oncol. Biol. Phys.* **84** 125–9

[7] Bujold A, Craig T, Jaffray D and Dawson L A 2012 Image-guided radiotherapy: has it influenced patient outcomes? *Semin. Radiat. Oncol.* **22** 50–61

[8] Winkel D *et al* 2019 Adaptive radiotherapy: the Elekta Unity MR-linac concept *Clin Transl Radiat Oncol* **18** 54–9

[9] Thureau S, Briens A, Decazes P, Castelli J, Barateau A, Garcia R, Thariat J and de Crevoisier R 2020 PET and MRI guided adaptive radiotherapy: rational, feasibility and benefit *Cancer Radiother* **24** 635–44

[10] Chen A M, Daly M E, Cui J, Mathai M, Benedict S and Purdy J A 2014 Clinical outcomes among patients with head and neck cancer treated by intensity-modulated radiotherapy with and without adaptive replanning *Head Neck* **36** 1541–6

[11] Henke L, Kashani R, Robinson C, Curcuru A, DeWees T, Bradley J, Green O, Michalski J, Mutic S and Parikh P J R 2018 Phase I trial of stereotactic MR-guided online adaptive radiation therapy (SMART) for the treatment of oligometastatic or unresectable primary malignancies of the abdomen *Radiother. Oncol.* **126** 519–26

[12] Bruynzeel A M, Tetar S U, Oei S S, Senan S, Haasbeek C J, Spoelstra F O, Piet A H, Meijnen P, van der Jagt M A B and Fraikin T J I J R O B P 2019 A prospective single-arm phase 2 study of stereotactic magnetic resonance guided adaptive radiation therapy for prostate cancer: early toxicity results *Int. J. Radiat. Oncol. Biol. Phys.* **105** 1086–94

[13] Hassanzadeh C, Rudra S, Bommireddy A, Hawkins W G, Wang-Gillam A, Fields R C, Cai B, Park J, Green O and Roach M J A I R O 2021 Ablative five-fraction stereotactic body radiation therapy for inoperable pancreatic cancer using online MR-guided adaptation *Adv. Radiat. Oncol.* **6** 100506

[14] Keall P, Poulsen P and Booth J T 2019 See, think, and act: real-time adaptive radiotherapy *Semin. Radiat. Oncol.* **29** 228–35

[15] Mutic S and Dempsey J F 2014 The ViewRay system: magnetic resonance–guided and controlled radiotherapy *Semin. Radiat. Oncol.* 196–99

[16] Raaymakers B, Jürgenliemk-Schulz I, Bol G, Glitzner M, Kotte A, Van Asselen B, De Boer J, Bluemink J, Hackett S and Moerland M J P M 2017 First patients treated with a 1.5 T MRI-Linac: clinical proof of concept of a high-precision, high-field MRI guided radiotherapy treatment *Phys. Med. Biol.* **62** L41

[17] Sibolt P, Andersson L M, Calmels L, Sjöström D, Bjelkengren U, Geertsen P and Behrens C F J P 2021 Clinical implementation of artificial intelligence-driven cone-beam computed tomography-guided online adaptive radiotherapy in the pelvic region *Phys. Imaging Radiat. Oncol.* **17** 1–7

[18] Bibault J E, Burgun A and Giraud P 2017 Artificial intelligence applied to radiation oncology *Cancer Radiother.* **21** 239–43

[19] Huynh E, Hosny A, Guthier C, Bitterman D S, Petit S F, Haas-Kogan D A, Kann B, Aerts H and Mak R H 2020 Artificial intelligence in radiation oncology *Nat. Rev. Clin. Oncol.* **17** 771–81

[20] Tseng H H, Luo Y, Cui S, Chien J T, Ten Haken R K and Naqa I E 2017 Deep reinforcement learning for automated radiation adaptation in lung cancer *Med. Phys.* **44** 6690–705

[21] Tseng H H, Luo Y, Ten Haken R K and El Naqa I 2018 The role of machine learning in knowledge-based response-adapted radiotherapy *Front. Oncol.* **8** 266

[22] Luk S M H, Meyer J, Young L A, Cao N, Ford E C, Phillips M H and Kalet A M 2019 Characterization of a Bayesian network-based radiotherapy plan verification model *Med. Phys.* **46** 2006–14

[23] Kalet A M, Luk S M H and Phillips M H 2020 Radiation therapy quality assurance tasks and tools: the many roles of machine learning *Med. Phys.* **47** e168–77

[24] Gopan O, Zeng J, Novak A, Nyflot M and Ford E 2016 The effectiveness of pretreatment physics plan review for detecting errors in radiation therapy *Med. Phys.* **43** 5181

[25] Ford E *et al* 2020 Strategies for effective physics plan and chart review in radiation therapy: report of AAPM Task Group 275 *Med. Phys.* **47** e236–72

[26] Rhee D J, Cardenas C E, Elhalawani H, McCarroll R, Zhang L, Yang J, Garden A S, Peterson C B, Beadle B M and Court L E J Mp 2019 Automatic detection of contouring errors using convolutional neural networks *Med. Phys.* **46** 5086–97

[27] Zhang J, Ates O and Li A 2016 Implementation of a machine learning-based automatic contour quality assurance tool for online adaptive radiation therapy of prostate cancer *Int. J. Radiat. Oncol.* **96** E668–68

[28] McIntosh C, Svistoun I and Purdie T G 2013 Groupwise conditional random forests for automatic shape classification and contour quality assessment in radiotherapy planning *IEEE Trans. Med. Imaging* **32** 1043–57

[29] Chen H C, Tan J, Dolly S, Kavanaugh J, Anastasio M A, Low D A, Harold Li H, Altman M, Gay H and Thorstad W L J Mp 2015 Automated contouring error detection based on supervised geometric attribute distribution models for radiation therapy: a general strategy *Med. Phys.* **42** 1048–59

[30] McCarroll R, Yang J, Cardenas C, Balter P, Burger H, Dalvie S, Kisling K, Mejia M, Naidoo K and Nelson C J M P 2017 Machine learning for the prediction of physician edits to clinical auto-contours in the head-and-neck: TU-FG-605-09 *Med. Phys.* **44**

[31] Azmandian F, Kaeli D, Dy J G, Hutchinson E, Ancukiewicz M, Niemierko A and Jiang S B 2007 Towards the development of an error checker for radiotherapy treatment plans: a preliminary study *Phys. Med. Biol.* **52** 6511–24

[32] Kalet A M, Gennari J H, Ford E C and Phillips M H 2015 Bayesian network models for error detection in radiotherapy plans *Phys. Med. Biol.* **60** 2735–49

[33] Moore K L *et al* 2015 Quantifying unnecessary normal tissue complication risks due to suboptimal planning: a secondary study of RTOG 0126 *Int. J. Radiat. Oncol.* **92** 228–35

[34] Shiraishi S, Tan J, Olsen L A and Moore K L 2015 Knowledge-based prediction of plan quality metrics in intracranial stereotactic radiosurgery *Med. Phys.* **42** 908

[35] Tol J P, Dahele M, Delaney A R, Slotman B J and Verbakel W F A R 2015 Can knowledge-based DVH predictions be used for automated, individualized quality assurance of radiotherapy treatment plans? *Radiat. Oncol.* **10**

[36] Pucchio A, Eisenhauer E A and Moraes F Y J N B 2021 Medical students need artificial intelligence and machine learning training *Nat. Biotechnol.* **39** 388–89

[37] Xing L, Goetsch S and Cai J J M P 2020 Artificial intelligence should be part of medical physics graduate program curriculum *Med. Phys.* **48** 1457–60

[38] French J and Chen L J J 2019 Preparing for artificial intelligence: systems-level implications for the medical imaging and radiation therapy professions *J. Med. Imaging Radiat. Sci.* **50** S20–23

[39] van Griethuysen J J M, Fedorov A, Parmar C, Hosny A, Aucoin N, Narayan V, Beets-Tan R G H, Fillion-Robin J C, Pieper S and Aerts H 2017 Computational radiomics system to decode the radiographic phenotype *Cancer Res.* **77** e104–07

[40] Zisserman K S A 2015 Very deep convolutional networks for large-scale image recognition *A Conf. Paper at ICLR 2015*

[41] Zisserman K S A 2014 A Very deep convolutional networks for large-scale image recognition arXiv: 1409.1556

[42] Cai B *et al* 2020 Evaluation and validation of artificial intelligence (AI) delineation models for CBCT-guided stereotactic online adaptive radiotherapy (STAR) targeting upper abdominal malignancies *Int. J. Radiat. Oncol. Biol. Phys.* **108** S43

[43] Kainz K, Lim S, Chen G-P and Allen Li X PreciseART™ adaptive radiation therapy software: dose monitoring, re-planning, and delivery verification https://www.accuray.com/wp-content/uploads/AP-PreciseART_Froedtert_WP-MKT000500.pdf

Chapter 8

AI-augmented image guidance for radiation therapy delivery

Zhao Wei

Image guidance enables the prescribed dose to be delivered to the target as planned while sparing the normal tissues. It is therefore of utmost importance for radiotherapy in clinical practice. Various imaging modalities have been employed as image guidance solutions. As an emerging processing tool for images, artificial intelligence (AI), especially deep convolutional networks, has been extensively used in these images heavily involved in guidance tasks. The AI tools have greatly augmented the accuracy of image guidance and simplified the workflow of clinical radiotherapy, for either interfraction or intrafraction motion. Specifical AI-based tasks include image registration, fiducial segmentation, real-time image reconstruction, image synthesis for magnetic resonance imaging-only radiotherapy.

8.1 Introduction to image guidance for radiotherapy

8.1.1 Background

It is well-known that radiotherapy is becoming increasingly conformal with the development of advanced beam delivery techniques and it is very important to make sure the patients are treated as planned. Routine radiotherapy assumes that anatomical alignment is consistent between the treatment planning CT (pCT) images and the actual anatomical morphology during beam delivery. However, this assumption is usually not achievable and the violation of the assumption has to be compensated using target margins. Although the margins can ensure the tumor to be irradiated with the prescribed dose, it also limits the conformity of radiotherapy and introduces irradiation to more normal tissues, which is not desirable, especially for steep dose gradient treatment. To tackle this limitation, image-guided radiotherapy (IGRT) which uses daily images to guide the treatment is routinely employed in practice [1, 2, 3]. IGRT ensures increased accuracy of dose delivery to the target

doi:10.1088/978-0-7503-3339-9ch8

volumes, as planned, and sparing the normal tissues. It is therefore a paradigm of modern radiotherapy [1, 2].

There are various image guidance methods for radiotherapy in clinical practice and these methods are based on different imaging modalities, such as x-ray imaging [3], ultrasonography (US) [4], optical imaging [5], magnetic resonance imaging [6] as well as electromagnetic transponder [7]. While the application of these methods relies on the specific treatment sites, different image modalities are able to be synergically used together to provide complementary guidance information to ensure better target localization before and during treatment. In general, the pretreatment guidance is a verification procedure for the fractionated beam delivery that makes the prescribed dose be delivered to the planning target volume (PTV). On the other hand, patients may undergo intrafraction motion (such as respiratory motion) during the beam delivery. The imaging modalities are able to monitor the motion in real-time and terminate the beam once the target is off-position with a predefined threshold. In addition, real-time motion management enables respiratory-gated treatment which significantly reduces the PTV for respiratory-involved radiotherapy [8].

Although these methods originated from photon therapy and are targeted to photon therapy, they can be translated to heavy-ion/proton therapy with the integration of additional monitoring and imaging equipment. However, due to the accuracy requirement differences between heavy-ion/proton therapy and photon therapy, in this chapter, we focus on image guidance for photon radiotherapy.

8.1.2 Current image guidance solutions

8.1.2.1 Infrared-based monitoring and surface imaging

Both infrared-based monitoring and surface monitoring are non-invasive techniques that can provide real-time image guidance without imposing additional radiation doses on the patient [9–11]. The infrared-based method uses passive infrared reflectors either mounted on the couch, a thermoplastic mask, the patient body, or a bite block, to provide the parameters of 6 degrees of freedom (DoF) of the target [12–14]. Specifically, the infrared reflectors which can be monitored by the stereoscopic in-room cameras are used to act as surrogates for the target position. The infrared-based methods therefore can be directly applied to intracranial stereotactic radiosurgery (SRS) which requires highly accurate treatment delivery [13].

Due to its capability of real-time monitoring, infrared reflectors can be used for motion management for extracranial sites. In this case, the infrared system is able to interrupt the beam irradiation during treatment once the target is beyond a predefined sub-millimeter threshold, and reposition the patient using a 6 DoF couch [13]. Compared to the fiducial-based invasive gold standard method, the non-invasive infrared-based methods can also be used for respiratory gating for lung, liver, and pancreas patients (or upper-abdomen cancer patients) [15, 16]. When compared with kilovoltage (kV) images of implanted clips, the infrared-based method has also reported a medical residual 3D setup error of 5.8 mm for breast treatment using multiple reflectors [17].

Since infrared reflectors are surrogates of the treatment target and cannot monitor the target position directly, they are usually used together with kV x-ray monitoring to reduce the internal–external correlation uncertainty. For example, on TrueBeam linac, the infrared-based respiratory gating system is used in conjunction with the on-board imager (OBI) where the kV imaging is used to verify the internal-target anatomy, and the beam delivery can be interrupted and the patient repositioned if the internal anatomy has changed [18].

Surface imaging uses high-definition optical cameras to map the patient's surface, which can be employed to monitor the patient motion in real-time. Specifically, the surface imaging system usually employs several room-mounted cameras to estimate the 6 DoF motion using projected light patterns [14]. During treatment, the real-time detected patient surface is compared with a reference surface which is reconstructed from the simulation CT. To enhance robustness, the translation and rotation of the patient is reported in real-time by registering several subsets (i.e., region-of-interest) of the surface with respect to the reference surface. The surface imaging-based approach mitigates the requirement of skin tattoos or invasive fixation devices for motion management [19]. In addition, this approach is also able to interrupt the beam delivery once the acquired real-time surface does not match the reference surface, and reposition the patient to the optimal match via the 6 DoFs feedback without using x-ray devices.

8.1.2.2 kV and MV x-ray imaging-based methods

X-ray imaging-based methods are routinely used for treatment verification and motion monitoring. For example, the kV x-ray imaging and the MV x-ray imaging are the standard practices for linacs and tomotherapy, respectively. These x-ray imaging-based methods are usually implemented in different hardware configurations, including standard linacs with an MV electronic portal imaging device (EPID) and a perpendicularly mounted kV imager system [20], and stereoscopic kV imaging using an orthogonal kV imaging system [21], as well as a real-time tracking radiotherapy (RTRT) system used with four kV imaging systems [8]. While monoscopic imaging is mainly used for patient setup, stereoscopic imaging and RTRT can not only be used for setup, but also for real-time motion management together with external breathing monitoring [22].

Due to poor soft-tissue contrast, high contrast fiducial markers are usually employed for x-ray imaging-based methods. The fiducials are implanted into or near the tumor and act as surrogates for the tumor position. In clinical practice, fiducial implantation has been widely used for liver cancer, prostate cancer, pancreatic cancer, and abdomen cancer patients [23]. For treatment setup or intrafraction motion monitoring, the fiducials can be segmented from the x-ray images automatically in real-time. Various segmentation methods have been proposed for either cylindrical or spherical markers or arbitrarily shaped markers. While the former can use simple parametric templates for fiducials segmentation [24], the latter usually requires complex templates [25]. For patient setup, the segmented fiducials are registered with fiducials in the pCT images, and the registration error suggests the misalignment between the treatment position and planning position. The patient is then repositioned according to the registration error. For respiratory-gated radiotherapy, the segmented fiducials are used to determine whether the treatment target are located at the specific inhale or exhale phase which is usually chosen for beam delivery [22].

Although fiducials implantation is able to provide highly accurate target positioning, its invasive nature introduces additional cost and prolonged treatment as it requires the availability of an interventional radiologist. In addition, a waiting time between implantation and pCT for fiducial stabilization may be needed. It also represents an added toxicity risk and complications [26] (including urinary tract infection for prostate and pneumothorax for lung) may be introduced after the implantation. Other limitations include fiducial migration and changes in the target position relative to the fiducials due to soft-tissue deformation, both of which suggest reduced targeting accuracy.

8.1.2.3 Stereoscopic imaging methods

Different from the 2D localization method, stereoscopic imaging is able to determine the target position via triangulation with high accuracy in real-time by using additional equipment. A typical implementation of stereoscopic imaging is the CyberKnife system which is originally developed for cranial radiosurgery back in 1990s [27]. Nowadays, the CyberKnife system has been extended to treat extracranial sites, including lung and spine cancer patients [28]. The system encompasses two ceiling-mounted kV x-ray sources, two opposed flat-panel detectors (FPD) which are mounted on the floor and a robotic 6 MV linac which is controlled via an automatic image processing console in real-time. Based on the live images acquired using the FPDs, the linac can realign the treatment beam via 6 DOF fashion. Specifically, intrafraction radiographs of the patient acquired using FPDs are registered to the digitally reconstructed radiographs (DRR) which are generated by forward projecting the pCT images using geometry consistent with the stereoscopic x-ray imaging system. Therefore, the system is able to monitor the target position and track the target during the beam delivery.

Shirato *et al* pioneered intra-treatment stereoscopic imaging by using an orthogonal in-room x-ray imaging system [8]. The imaging part which consists of four x-ray sources on the floor and four corresponding ceiling-mounted detectors, was installed together with a conventional linac to make up the RTRT system. Instead of tracking the tumor with the treatment beam, the treatment was performed in a gated fashion and gating was triggered via real-time position of the fiducials acquired using the stereoscopic imaging system. Specifically, the beam pulse and the fiducial positions were synchronized such that the beam is delivered only when the fiducials were within a predefined threshold [29]. Different from the CyberKnife system, the RTRT system is able to perform high-frequency image acquisition and a total of thirty kV image pairs can be acquired per second. The high monitoring rate has enabled the system to be applied to various treatment sites [30, 31].

8.1.2.4 Magnetic resonance imaging

Magnetic resonance imaging (MRI) scanners employ strong magnetic fields, magnetic field gradients, and radio waves to generate images of anatomy and the physiological processes of the body. MRI has been widely used in hospitals and clinics for disease diagnosis, staging and follow-up. In radiotherapy, magnetic resonance-guided radiation therapy (MRgRT) combines a magnetic resonance imaging unit with a radiation therapy unit, allowing real-time imaging of target volumes and organs at risk before and during treatment delivery with replanning as necessary, which is particularly useful in sites affected by inter- and intrafraction motion such as the thorax, abdomen, and pelvis [32]. Compared to daily cone-beam computed tomography (CBCT) which is used for pretreatment patient setup, MRI can provide significantly improved soft-tissue visualization for IGRT and adaptive radiotherapy (ART).

Several MRgRT systems with various implementation stages and characteristics have been developed in the past decade. The first MRgRT system used in clinical practice was the MRIdian system which was released by ViewRay [33]. The MRIdian system originally encompasses a tri-cobalt 60 source and a 0.35 T MRI. The system was upgraded by replacing the cobalt source with a 6 MV flattening filter free (FFF) linac to enhance beam penetration and dose uniformity in 2018. The upgraded system is also able to decrease penumbra and surface dose, therefore sparing the normal tissue at the surface. Meanwhile, Elekta and Phillips have incorporated a 7 MV FFF linac together with a 1.5 T MRI [34], and the new system (named Unity) has been installed in at least seven institutions in Europe and USA. The Unity delivered the first treatment at the UMC Utrecht in 2017, and later at Royal Marsden Hospital and at the Christie in 2018 and in 2019, respectively.

8.1.2.5 Ultrasound imaging

Although on-board x-ray imaging has been the standard practice in radiotherapy for a long time, advanced radiotherapy techniques such as ART, require an image modality which has superior soft-tissue contrast such that the treatment target can be imaged directly. With the increasing use of hypofractionated radiotherapy treatment regimens, such as stereotactic ablative radiotherapy (SABR), the role of inter-fractional and intrafractional imaging technologies is becoming more and more important to ensure safe and effective beam delivery. Ultrasound (US)-based imaging techniques are able to provide non-invasive, marker-free, and real-time volumetric images. Without using ionizing radiation, US offers superior soft-tissue contrast, outperforming classical x-ray or CT-based guidance techniques. This merit makes US-based guidance be suitable for abdominal and pelvic soft-tissue tumor sites, especially for the liver, pancreas, and prostate. In practice, there have been commercialized inter-fractional US guidance systems for pretreatment patient positioning and verification [4, 35]. The first US-based guidance system (B-Mode Acquisition and Targeting (BAT) system) for inter-fractional imaging was introduced in the late 1990s [36]. The system tracks the position of the US probe with respect to the linac by using a 2D diagnostic US imaging system together with an optical solution.

By integrating with existing linacs, US guidance systems offer real-time, volumetric, and marker-free target tracking for intrafractional motion management during beam delivery. The intrafractional US guidance systems encompass a hardware device to make sure the US probe in the imaging position during therapy, and real-time US images were transferred outside the treatment room. While avoiding possible interference with the patient's body, the linac, and treatment beams, the device (possibly a robotic hardware) can hold the US probe to maintain the treatment target within the field of view of the US imaging system throughout beam delivery. The Clarity Autoscan System which was the first US guidance system for intrafractional imaging is a fixture that is mounted to a plate on the couch and manually operates in 5-DOF [37]. The US probe is locked into the imaging position by the fixture which is remotely controlled by the sonographer who is outside the treatment room during beam delivery. Without physically moving the US probe head, the 3D/4D probe is able to automatically acquire volumetric US images. With the geometry of the fixture and US probe, the whole imaging system is set up in a transperineal way such that all system hardware is out of the delivery plane of the linacs. The guidance system is therefore not able to interfere with the radiation treatment procedure and also enables simultaneous CBCT/US imaging during the pretreatment patient setup phase [38].

8.1.2.6 Tomosynthesis imaging

Although conventionally used for digital chest and mammography, digital tomosynthesis (DTS) has been proposed as a new paradigm for radiation treatment verification recently and real-time guidance of treatment. DTS acquires x-ray projections in a limited rotation angle range (usually $\pm 15°$) and performs limited-angle tomography which has a comparable in-plane resolution to that of full-field digital mammography, and inferior out-of-plane resolution. Due to partial data sampling with incomplete projections, iterative image reconstruction algorithms (such as expectation maximization algorithms) can yield superior image quality compared to the classical filtered projection algorithm which requires a complete set of data. On the other hand, due to the limited gantry rotation, the radiation dose and imaging time are substantially reduced compared to conventional full angle rotation CT scans [39].

As an alternative to the standard CBCT technique, both DTS with an on-board kV imager (kV-DTS) and megavoltage (MV-DTS) beam has been proposed for IGRT. The feasibility of pretreatment target localization using kV-DTS has been demonstrated for different patient sites, including prostate, head-and-neck, and liver [39, 40]. Compared to either kV or MV radiographs, kV-DTS yields substantially more anatomic information. Meanwhile, due to the reduced image acquisition time, breath-hold DTS can be performed to mitigate respiratory motion artifacts. The feasibility of performing MV-DTS has also been demonstrated clinically in the treatment room for IGRT [41]. A phantom study has shown that MV-DTS has the same signal-difference-to-noise ratio as MV-CBCT for the same scanning dose. Although having an inferior spatial resolution in the direction perpendicular to the plane of reconstruction, MV-DTS has a better spatial resolution in the reconstruction planes. Prostate patients results also show comparable tissue contrast between MV-DTS and MV-CBCT.

Since DTS only acquires x-ray projections in a limited-angle range, it has an anisotropic spatial resolution. In order to improve the spatial resolution, DTS

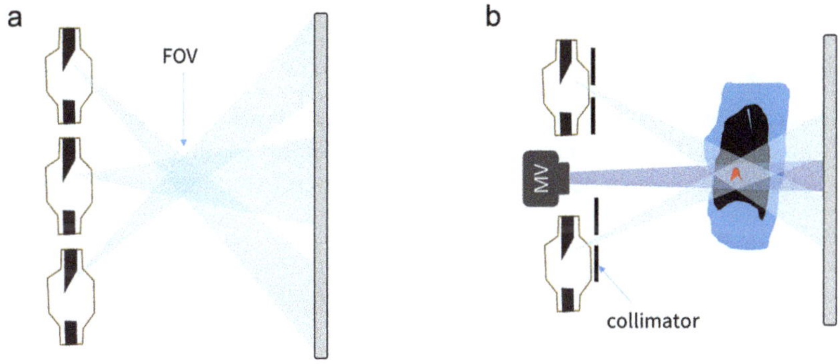

Figure 8.1. (a) Tomosynthesis design using multiple sources for parallel data acquisition. (b) Side view of the system, x-ray tubes are installed around the treatment head, and the kV x-ray photons are collimated down to the isocenter. Adapted from [43] John Wiley & Sons. Copyright 2017 American Association of Physicists in Medicine.

images acquired using on-board devices can be performed in two angular ranges separated by 90°. By integrating the two sets of DTS images, the resulting images (named IDTS) are able to take advantage of both DTS images which have a complementary spatial resolution in orthogonal planes, yielding high spatial resolution in both coronal and sagittal planes [42].

DTS can not only be used for pretreatment verification, it can also be used for real-time guidance of radiation therapy. Different from previous tomosynthesis designs which acquire limited angular projections and have temporal resolution on the order of seconds. A novel tomosynthesis design uses multiple sources to enable parallel data acquisition, as shown in figure 8.1. Specifically, the field of view is illuminated simultaneously with multiple sources and the temporal resolution of the design is up to 30 frames per second. The feasibility of real-time guidance using the novel design has been demonstrated using simulated lung tumor data. In practice, scanning beam digital x-ray (SBDX) is one implementation capable of real-time tomosynthesis. However, SBDX requires considerable hardware and has not been commercially used until now [43].

8.1.3 AI tools and networks for image guidance

Artificial intelligence (AI) is a very general concept and can also be called machine intelligence. It encompasses classical machine learning approaches (such as K-mean clustering) and the emerging deep learning approaches (such as convolutional neural network). Table 8.1 shows typical approaches in machine learning and deep learning. Classical machine learning approaches rely on human-engineered features and have achieved varying degrees of clinical utility. While these features (such as size, diameter, gray values, etc) are generally interpretable, the feature extraction procedure is usually time-consuming and accurate feature engineering requires careful feature selection and loop iterations, which limit the application of machine learning approaches in routine practice [44].

Table 8.1. Typical approaches in machine learning and deep learning.

Machine learning	Deep learning
Support-vector machines (SVM), principal component analysis (PCA), manifold learning, regression analysis, decision trees	Convolutional neural network (CNN), reinforcement learning, generative adversarial networks (GAN), recurrent neural networks (RNN)

Deep learning tools are able to automatically extract features using large scale deep neural networks. Although often at a cost of feature interpretability, deep neural networks provide a large learning capacity and are therefore able to find complex, nonlinear relationships in training data. With the rapidly increasing large amounts of data available and computational power, deep learning-based AI tools have become emerging techniques in radiation oncology, especially in image-based tasks (such as IGRT) and deep learning-based approaches (such as CNN) are extremely suitable for these tasks.

For the task of image guidance in radiotherapy, both machine learning and deep learning-based approaches have been employed. In the gated lung cancer treatment, the gating signal can be treated as a classification task where the beam ON and OFF corresponds to two classes. In this case, either classical machine learning algorithms or deep learning algorithms which are suitable for classification (including PCA, CNN) have been evaluated for gated lung cancer radiotherapy [45]. For inter-fractional and intrafractional motion monitoring, deep neural networks for object detection (such as Faster R-CNN, Mask R-CNN) can be used for pretreatment patient setup and real-time target localization during treatment. Since image guidance relies heavily on the implanted markers, CNN-based needle and fiducial segmentation approaches have also been extensively investigated [46]. 3D Image registration between pretreatment CBCT and pCT as well as 2D/3D image registration between kV images and pCT images play an important role in image guidance. While there are a huge number of classical image registration methods, deep learning-based image registration has also been extensively studied for image guidance. Popular deep neural networks for image guidance include reinforcement learning [47], GANs [48], and unsupervised CNNs [49, 50].

8.2 Image guidance for interfraction motion

8.2.1 Patients setup based on orthogonal kV images

8.2.1.1 Classical fiducial matching

For lung tumors treated in free-breathing, the size of the PTV can be substantial if the internal-target-volume (ITV) concept is used since this comprises the tumor position in all phases of the breathing cycle with an extra margin. Respiratory-gated lung cancer radiotherapy holds promise to precisely deliver the prescribed radiation dose to the tumor, while minimizing the incidence and severity of normal tissue

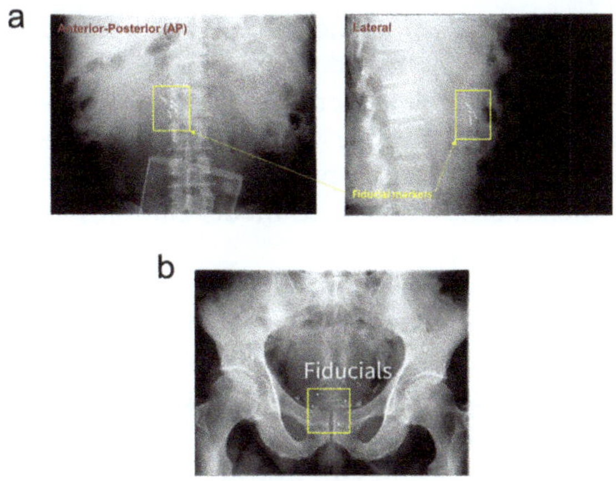

Figure 8.2. Implanted gold fiducial markers used for daily patient setup and real-time tracking in pancreatic (a) and prostate (b) IGRT. Reprinted with permission from [58], copyright (2019), with permission from Elsevier.

complications. Respiratory gating limits radiation exposure to a portion of the breathing cycle when the tumor is in a predefined gating window, and the gating mechanism often relies on implanted fiducials [8, 23, 29].

Fiducials are also useful for prostate cancer patients and pancreatic cancer patients, as shown in figure 8.2. Prostate cancer patients are usually set up based on the fiducial markers which are implanted inside the prostate gland before treatment planning. Specifically, the daily images are registered with the planning images to correct the interfractional motion. Studies have shown the precision of patient set up based on fiducials is superior to that based on patient anatomy (such as bony structures), and the use of fiducials is an effective way to spare normal tissues [51, 53]. Different from prostate cancer treatment, pancreatic cancer treatment is much more challenging due to the respiratory motion. The fiducials are therefore ideal surrogates for better target localization. Clinical studies using fiducials in advanced pancreatic cancer patients show excellent tumor local control probability [54].

8.2.1.2 Deep learning-based fiducial-free setup

Although fiducials have achieved accurate target localization, the implantation process is invasive and requires an interventional procedure which prolongs the treatment workflow. In addition, the fiducials may cause complications to patients and also introduce artifacts in the planning images which are undesirable for treatment planning.

Deep learning uses hierarchical neural networks to extract features from training data and incorporate prior knowledge into a predictive model. Deep learning-based image analysis of monoscopic or stereoscopic kV x-ray image(s) acquired before treatment delivery has potential to provide information about the position of the tumor target. To this end, pretreatment CT simulations were usually employed to develop the data-driven deep learning models [57, 58]. Specifically, the model learns multiple levels of representations that correspond to different levels of abstraction from the input x-ray images to perform predictions. For a case such as target localization for patient setup, a large amount of annotated training dataset is generated using the CT simulations to train the deep learning model, and the model is patient-specific which means the trained model can only be used for the patient during treatment.

Since model training usually requires a large amount of kV projections and it is not possible to acquire these data directly from the patient. To generate kV projection x-ray images that reflect the realistic treatment scenarios, motion vector fields (MVFs) generated by registering the pCT images and the daily CBCT images are employed to deform the pretreatment pCT. The deformed pCT is then augmented by rotation and translation procedure to further enlarge the number of training samples. The resulting CT images are then used to generate digitally reconstructed radiographs (DRRs) using the geometry of the on-board imager system. In addition to the CT images, the planning target volume (PTV) associated with the pCT images is also computationally projected on the virtual imager to yield a PTV-only radiograph. The position of the PTV is calculated and attached to the corresponding DRR to make up an annotated training sample. By randomly combining the MVFs, thousands of annotated samples can be generated to train the patient-specific target localization deep neural network which can be used for subsequent target localization, as shown in figure 8.3. Evaluation studies using testing samples not seen in the training phase show the model achieve a target localization accuracy of 3 mm for pancreatic tumor [59].

Of note, the integration of pCT prior knowledge and its realistic deformations into deep convolutional features enables the trained model to visualize the target in the x-ray image that would otherwise be invisible to the human eye [60]. More importantly, different from current clinical practice, the approach does not rely on implanted fiducials for target localization. The deep learning-based fiducial-free target localization methods have successfully applied to prostate cancer patients [60], pancreatic cancer patients who treated with linacs [61], and patients who received spinal stereotactic radiosurgery [62].

8.2.2 Pretreatment daily cone-beam CT imaging

8.2.2.1 Image registration based on bony structures and soft tissues

Cone-beam computed tomography (CBCT) based on a kV imaging system capable of radiography, fluoroscopy has been integrated with a medical linear accelerator. The kV imaging system consists of an x-ray tube and a flat-panel detector. Projection measurements from different view angles are acquired during the gantry rotates around the patient couch. Volumetric images are reconstructed using either classical filtered backprojection or iterative image reconstruction algorithms [63, 64].

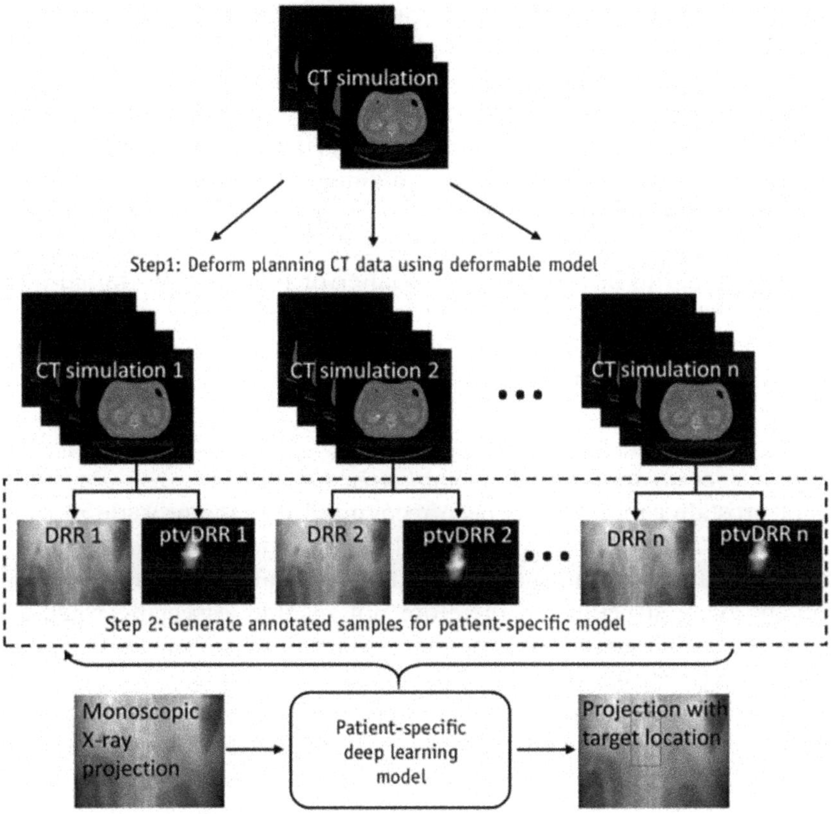

Figure 8.3. Deep learning-based fiducial-free target localization method. Abbreviations: CT = computed tomography; DRR = digitally reconstructed radiograph; ptvDRR = planning target volume-only digitally reconstructed radiograph. Reprinted with permission from [58], copyright (2019), with permission from Elsevier.

In the context of image guidance using CBCT, In the intended image guidance model for cone-beam CT, fraction-by-fraction repositioning will be achieved by therapist-driven registration of the CBCT image to the CT-defined CTV. The registration algorithm allows for corrections in the three translational and three rotational dimensions. The decision to use either soft-tissue (gray) matching versus bony target registration was determined by technical and clinical factors. Usually, registration using bony structures was considered to be a more robust algorithm and efficient.

For the treatment of stereotactic or hypofractionated lung radiotherapy (i.e., stereotactic body radiotherapy (SBRT)), a CBCT scan is performed using on-board imager before each treatment fraction. The CBCT images are then registered to the pCT images with respect to the tumor volumes. This procedure is a normalized cross-correlation match and setup error can be calculated for the superior-inferior (SI), anterior-posterior (AP), and left-right (LR) directions.

For the treatment of stereotactic or hypofractionated lung radiotherapy (i.e., stereotactic body radiotherapy (SBRT)), a CBCT scan is performed using on-board imager before each treatment fraction. The CBCT images are then registered to the pCT images with respect to the tumor volumes. This procedure is a normalized cross-correlation match and setup error can be calculated for the superior-inferior (SI), anterior-posterior (AP), and left-right (LR) directions. In addition, a second CBCT was acquired to measure any residual error following the initial correction, confirming the accuracy of the target position. If the residual (postcorrectional) error was $\leqslant$2 mm in all three directions, the patient was treated in the corrected position. If the residual error was >2 mm, additional corrections were performed until a residual $\leqslant$2 mm was achieved [66].

8.2.2.2 Image registration based on implanted fiducials

In cases of prostate cancer, it has been recognized that the prostate is a moveable structure and the nature of its motion is well-documented. For prostate target, bony anatomy is not a strong surrogate for a daily prostate position. The registration based on the bony structures is therefore not reliable, especially when the daily CBCT images are suffering from various artifacts and are not suitable for image registration using soft tissues [3].

In many institutes, the standard of care has been to implant fiducial markers that can be visualized on orthogonal kV images and used as surrogates for target positioning. Because implanting fiducials before initiating treatment is not without risk, it would be useful to accurately localize the target on a daily basis without necessitating such a procedure. In this scenario, CBCT images were obtained by use of standard dose technique (125 kV, 80 mA, 25 milliseconds) and on-board imager before the treatments. The fiducials on CBCT images were then co-registered with the fiducials on the reference CT images. This process can be achieved using both automatic alignments with gray value-based registration and manual alignment to the fiducials. Studies have shown alignment based on fiducials for prostate IGRT is superior to CBCT image registration using soft-tissue [67, 68], and daily alignment using CBCT fiducial images is one of the most reliable methods to maintain accuracy in prostate IGRT.

However, compared to soft-tissue CBCT, the benefits of the use of fiducials together with daily CBCT are still unclear. Yildirim *et al* compared fiducial-based CBCT (CBCT-FM) image guided radiotherapy and soft-tissue cone-beam computed tomography (CBCT-P) in prostate cancer patients. For each patient, both CBCT-FM and CBCT-P were employed for alignment. The results show no difference in median displacement was found between CBCT-P and CBCT-FM. Meanwhile, the displacements in all three directions determined by CBCT-P and CBCT-FM were strongly positively correlated with each other. For prostate cancer patients, the CBCT-FM did not show superior performance to the CBCT-FM for IGRT [69].

8.3 Image guidance for intrafraction motion

8.3.1 Real-time monitoring methods

8.3.1.1 Fiducial-based real-time tracking radiotherapy

Real-time motion monitoring or tracking relies heavily on fiducials. For those technologies including kV, MV, combined kV/MV, and electromagnetic methods, fiducials have been implanted into sites such as the prostate, lung, liver, and pancreas for intrafraction motion monitoring. These technologies have been integrated into various online solutions which include CyberKnife (Accuray) [27], ExacTrac (Brainlab) [14], Vero (Brainlab and Mitsubishi) [70], COSMIK [71], KIM [72], Calypso (Varian) [73].

The CyberKnife® system was originally developed to deliver stereotactic radiosurgery (SRS) for cranial tumor patients in the 1990s [27]. Shortly thereafter, it was modified to treat extracranial sites, such as the spinal cord and lungs [28]. By using two ceiling-mounted kV sources together with two opposed floor-mounted flat-panel detectors, and a robotic 6 MV-linac controlled by automatic image processing software, CyberKnife is the first radiotherapy machine that is able to perform real-time motion monitoring and tracking simultaneously. The treatment beam can be realigned with 6 DOFs in a non-isocenter manner by using the robotic linac.

The ExacTrac system uses a combined optical and x-ray imaging system for image guidance [73]. Specifically, ceiling-mounted cameras detect the infrared (IR) signals reflected by five to seven reflective markers placed on the patient. An IR reflector is also placed on the couch to automatically adjust the couch. The IR signals are able to reflect respiratory motion. During treatment, paired x-ray images are acquired when the external IR signals match the predefined gating threshold. Based on the x-ray images, 3D triangulated positions of fiducials are compared with the reference positions. In case the discrepancy between the reference positions and triangulated positions are larger than a set tolerance, the radiation beam is switched off and the patient is realigned.

The Vero system is another optical IR and x-ray imaging combined system [70]. Before the treatment, an external correlation model (ECM) is built using stereoscopic kV imaging (at 11 Hz) data and external IR (at 50 Hz) monitoring data acquired in a 20–40 s training session. With the trained ECM, the target position is predicted in real-time during the whole treatment procedure with a 2 s interval. The predicted target position is associated with a tolerance region with 3 mm radius, and the clinicians can terminate the beam delivery if the tolerance is systematically exceeded.

Without the use of radiation dose, electromagnetic systems are able to localize implanted transponders or transmitters in 3D and real-time. Calypso (Varian Medical Systems) is the most commonly used system with electromagnetic resonance circuits sealed in a glass capsule [74]. In clinical practice, three transponders with resonance frequencies from 300 kHz to 500 kHz are usually implanted into the tumor target or adjacent normal tissue. The transponders are excited one by one by an array of excitation coils in a panel above the patient. By using triangulation, a second array of receiver coils is used to localize the resonating transponder. As a result, the 3D position of the transponder centroid can be determined with a frequency of 10–25 Hz. Meanwhile, IR markers on the panel are tracked by three room-mounted cameras to determine the position relative to the accelerator iso-center. Note that the beam depth dose curves and beam attenuation can be changed by the antenna panel, but studies have shown the consequential dosimetric impact on treatment plans is marginal.

8.3.1.2 kV monoscopic imaging

The on-board kV imaging system is installed perpendicularly to the MV treatment head on a standard linac. Due to the limited 2D projection, the motion in 3D is usually inferred using advanced algorithms together with prior knowledge. Based on the projection theory, a target projected onto an imager suggests the target is located somewhere on the propagation path of the ray between the x-ray source and the projection. By establishing a model (such as respiratory phase correlated model) that allows estimation of the target position beyond the ray path, real-time monoscopic target localization in 3D is possible. For example, a motion predictive model can be trained using kV images acquired before treatment and the motion during treatment is therefore predicted using the model and real-time kV images. In addition, compared to MV images, the better contrast provided by kV images enables more reliable detection of treatment targets (fiducials or tumor).

For simplicity, the motion taking place beyond the ray path can be neglected. By using the position of the path ray of a training image that is the closest to the path ray of the current image frame, the real-time 3D target position is then determined by triangulation. The triangulation is the backbone of Sequential Stereo (Varian Medical System) technology which was adopted by online 3D spine target monitoring during SABR delivery [75]. In practice, several training images whose path rays are within a predefined threshold distance from the path ray of the current image can be included in triangulation with different weights.

Another approach is to use the probability density function (PDF) for the target position prediction. The 3D PDF can be derived from a sequence of training images. Real-time target position is therefore estimated as the expectation of the PDF along the path ray. An example is to use spatial probability density to estimate prostate position with a single x-ray projection [76]. By integrating template-based fiducial segmentation and the Gaussian PDF method, kV Intrafraction Monitoring (KIM) has been employed both retrospectively [77] and prospectively [72] to estimate 3D motion for prostate cancer patients. Similar methods have also been used in VMAT liver tumor treatment [78] and pancreatic tumor [79] in daily CBCT for intrafraction motion estimation. The tumor location in these clinical applications is calculated based on the position of the implanted fiducials. The accuracy of KIM has been assessed with respect to post-treatment triangulation and submillimetre accuracy has been reported in retrospective analysis [80] as well as prospective motion monitoring with beam gating and couch-shifts [81]. In addition, the KIM system has also been extended to monitor 6 DOFs motion for prostate targets [82]. Submillimetre and sub-degree accuracy of prostate and lung tumors motion management have been achieved in phantom studies [83]. As an alternative to KIM, hybrid monitoring using combined optical and sparse monoscopic imaging with kV x-rays (COSMIK) has also been implemented on standard linacs [71].

As a major contribution to AI, machine learning-based approaches have also been studied for markerless IGRT based on kV monoscopic imaging. For gated lung cancer radiotherapy, the gating signal can be modeled as a binary pattern classification task, which is a typical machine learning problem and can be performed using a combined support-vector machine (SVM) and principal component analysis (PCA) [45]. In addition, the classification task can also be solved using combined machine learning methods (artificial neural networks-ANN and SVM) and dimensionality reduction techniques (PCA and four nonlinear manifold learning methods). Evaluation studies using lung cancer patients show PCA combined with either machine learning methods achieved a better performance than nonlinear manifold learning methods, and ANN combined with PCA achieve the best performance for gated radiotherapy in terms of classification accuracy and recall rate.

8.3.1.3 MV monoscopic imaging

The treatment beam itself can provide MV imaging together with an electronic portal imaging device (EPID). This imaging modality uses treatment dose and provides monoscopic imaging in the beam's eye view (BEV). Although it is 2D imaging, MV monoscopic imaging can show motion perpendicular to the treatment beam which is most sensitive to dose delivery in the photon radiotherapy scenario, and it can be performed both with and without fiducials. Figure 8.4 shows tumor visibility for lung cancer patients using MV imaging. The results show there is no relationship between tumor location and visibility. However, compared to kV imaging, MV imaging yields inferior soft-tissue contrast and its field of view is limited to and affected by the multi-leaf collimator.

Based on MV imaging of four implanted fiducials, Deutschmann *et al* pioneered the work of estimation of the positional and rotational pose prostate which are employed to adapt the treatment [84]. Specifically, without adjusting the patient couch, each segment for IMRT treatment can be adjusted according to the prostate position determined before this specific segment. To ensure the accuracy of the beam delivery, the positions of the target as well as the segment parameters were recorded and verified in the treatment planning system. More than 1000 fractions of 39 patients who underwent prostate IMRT were respectively studied using the method. The results show mitigation larger than 2 mm and a rotation of larger than 12 degrees for the prostate have been observed in 82% of the fractions and 10% of the fractions, respectively. Therefore, safe margin reduction can be enabled by interfraction and intrafraction motion measurements and adaption. In addition to the 2D motion measurement via BEV, real-time 3D target position can be calculated using the motion measured with clinical MV prostate image together with a 2D to 3D trajectory reconstruction algorithm. With MLC tracking, the feasibility of motion monitoring using MV BEV was demonstrated for SBRT delivery in pigs [85]. During this experimental implementation, the motion estimation was based on the implanted stent in the lung region. However, studies also show fiducial-free motion monitoring was also achievable on clinically acquired lung MV monoscopic images [86–88]. An example of tumor tracking using EPID is shown in figure 8.5.

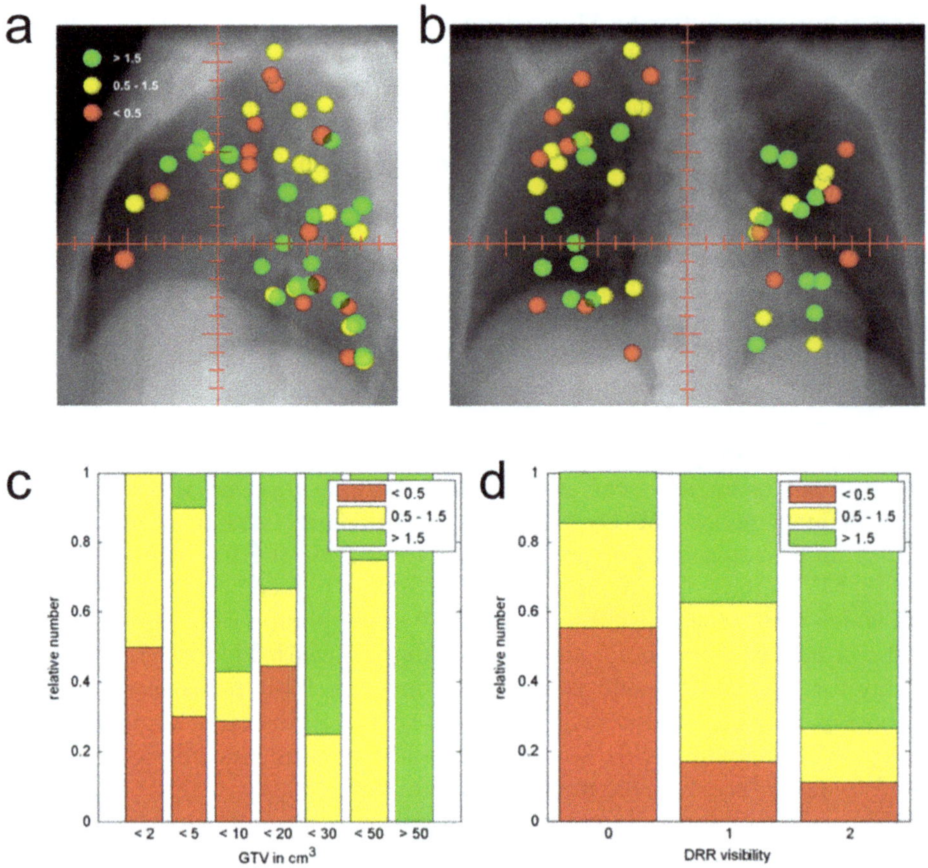

Figure 8.4. The relationship between tumor visibility and tumor location. The green (visibility > 1.5), yellow (0.5 < visibility < 1.5), and red (visibility < 0.5) colors show the mean rating for the tumor visibility by three independent observers. Tumor visibility of the MV imaging of 49 tumors in (a) left-right and (b) anterior–posterior planes. Dependences on (c) GTV and (d) DRR visibility, respectively. Reprinted with permission from [86], copyright (2009), with permission from Elsevier.

8.3.2 Real-time needle and fiducial segmentation

8.3.2.1 Deep learning-based methods

Most real-time image guided systems rely heavily on the accurate and efficient segmentation of implanted fiducial markers in each image to resolve the 3D motion based on 2D images, such as the MV monoscopic imaging [84, 85] in the previous subsection. Deep learning-based image segmentation has been extensively investigated in recent years. For the purpose of real-time fiducial segmentation, Mylonas *et al* propose an automatic deep learning-based framework for the tracking of arbitrarily shaped markers in fluoroscopic images without prior knowledge of the marker properties. In order to provide annotated data for model training, they created several datasets from phantom and patient fluoroscopic images to be used for the training and validation of different CNN models. For the outlined problem,

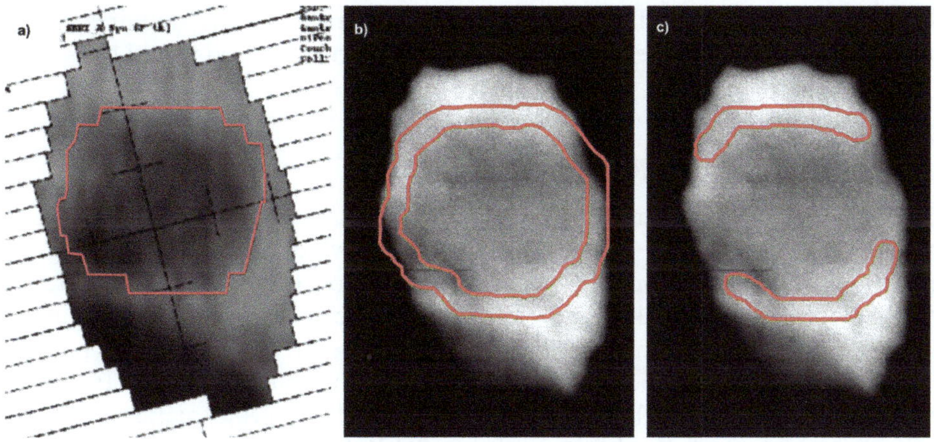

Figure 8.5. Tumor tracking using an electronic portal imaging device (EPID) with overlaid DRR image. (a) Example of a DRR with overlaid tumor contour. (b) Corresponding image acquired using EPID with tumor mask generated using DRR. (c) Modified mask for real-time tumor tracking. Reprinted with permission from [86], copyright (2009), with permission from Elsevier.

the CNNs are binary classifiers to differentiate between positive and negative sub-images (marker versus background). In addition, the effects of transfer learning and adding more noisy data into the training datasets for data augmentation are employed. Testing results on cylindrical shaped markers and then arbitrarily shaped markers (coiled) show high classification performances on unseen patient images during training phase were achieved with the deep learning approach. In addition, by using a simple tracking system, the CNN models are able to monitor intra-fraction motion without prior knowledge about the marker properties [46].

8.3.2.2 Comparison with classical methods

Instead of deep learning-based approaches, many current segmentation methods are based on template matching which requires prior information about the marker. A dynamic programming approach is used together with the template matching to track the markers with high sensitivity [89]. When regular shaped markers (e.g. spherical fiducials) are used, their properties (such as dimensions) can be used to build the template. However, regular shaped markers are more likely to be suffered from migration. Arbitrarily shaped markers, such as coiled markers, are able to decrease migration, but their properties are difficult to be used to build the template. In this case, an additional learning process can be employed to determine the marker properties and a template can be built based on the learned properties. Regmi *et al* developed a semi-automated method to construct the marker templates from pCT images. However, the markers are usually associated with metal artifacts in most kV CT images. Of note, templates constructed using kV images acquired prior to the treatment are not reliable and online MV images are therefore usually used to build the templates prior to beam delivery. Of note, the learning process requires additional projection measurements, which means patients are subjected to additional imaging dose. To address these issues, a system that requires no prior knowledge of marker properties or an additional learning period would be beneficial to the patients [46].

8.4 Real-time 3D IGRT on standard linac

IGRT has been routinely implemented on standard linacs with implanted fiducials in real-time 2D fashion. This 2D guidance technique which enables monitoring while beam treatment is a major step forward in radiation oncology. It can detect the intrafraction motion and take appropriate action which usually triggers a 3D imaging acquisition and a consequence couch correction if necessary. However, this procedure prolongs the treatment process and also suffers from limited accuracy. In addition, advanced applications including MLC tracking, dose reconstruction and couch tracking cannot be performed using real-time 2D IGRT. To overcome the limitations of the routinely used real-time 2D IGRT regime while taking advantage of its widespread availability, the ideal solution is to perform 3D IGRT with standard linacs by using advanced algorithms (such as machine learning-based algorithms). In the following section, we introduce several machine learning-based volumetric reconstruction techniques using a single projection view data for real-time 3D IGRT.

For lung and upper-abdomen (such as liver and pancreas) cancer patients, the respiratory motion can be modeled using principal component analysis (PCA) which provides the best linear representation of the 4D dynamic data. The PCA motion model imposes inherent regularization on the representation and voxels move similarly therefore have similar PCA representations [90]. Based on this principle, Li *et al* developed a real-time volumetric image reconstruction and 3D tumor localization method for lung cancer radiotherapy by using a single x-ray projection, as shown in figure 8.3. Specifically, deformation vector fields (DVFs) between phase-resolved 4D-CT images can be represented by a few PCA eigenvectors and coefficients. To reconstruct real-time volumetric images, DVFs generated by updating the PCA coefficients were applied to the reference pCT images to yield new volumetric images, which were used to compute digitally projection to match the measured single-view projection. This procedure was iteratively optimized such that the *l*2-norm between the measured and calculated projections was minimized. Evaluation studies using both dynamic numerical phantom data and clinical lung cancer patients show average 3D tumor localization errors of 0.8 ± 0.5 and below 2 mm were achieved, respectively [91].

Due to their powerful ability to learn complex relationships and to incorporate prior knowledge into a predictive model via feature extraction and representation learning, deep neural networks were also used to reconstruct real-time volumetric CT images for IGRT [92]. To this end, the image reconstruction procedure is formulated as a feature-space transformation between a single-view 2D projection and a 3D volumetric image within a representation-generation (encoding-decoding) framework. A residual block-based representation network was developed to encode projection measurement, yielding a high-level representation tensor, which was then reshaped by a transformation module. With the transformed tensor, 3D volumetric reconstruction was performed subsequently using a generation network. The representation network, the transformation module, and the generation network were synergetically trained together using patient pCT images or phase-resolved 4D-CT data. The feasibility of the deep learning-based volumetric reconstruction approach was demonstrated using upper-abdomen, lung, and head-and-neck CT scans. The results show the approach provides high performance volumetric anatomical images by using only a single-view projection as input for the trained model [92]. The real-time volumetric images provide a direct solution for 3D IGRT.

Different from classical volumetric CT reconstruction, which needs complete projection data required by Shannon–Nyquist theorem and Tuy condition [93, 94], deep learning-based image reconstruction is able to the push sparse projection sampling to the limit of a single view by taking advantage of the prior patient anatomical information. It is therefore possible to use the real-time monoscopic kV image acquired during beam delivery to reconstruct volumetric images for 3D IGRT. This study provides a framework for ultra-sparse CT image reconstruction via deep learning approaches. While classical machine learning-based volumetric reconstruction methods can only be applied to respiratory-involved image reconstruction with the respiratory modeled by 4D CT, the deep learning-based method is more general and can be applied to more treatment sites and clinical applications (such as head-and-neck patients) [92].

Based on Shen *et al* pioneering work on deep learning-based ultra-sparse image reconstruction, a novel generative adversarial network-based method was proposed to derive instantaneous volumetric images from a single 2D projection with perceptual supervision [95]. Like previous work, the network consists of encoding, transformation and decoding modules. Instead of using an image distance loss between the predicted images and the ground truth images, and feature space-based perceptual loss is introduced and integrated into the loss function. The results show the new loss function enables a mass distance error within 2.6 mm, and the method can yield acceptable results for challenging scenarios where increased respiratory motion amplitude and tumor shrinkage are present [95].

8.5 Summary

Various image guidance methods have been implemented in clinical practice for radiotherapy. These methods have made strides to deliver more conformal therapeutic beam delivery to the treatment target while sparing normal tissues. AI developments on image guidance technologies, which range from kV and MV modalities to 2D and 3D techniques, from intrefraction to intrafraction, from x-ray to MRI, and eventually to ultrasound and tomosynthesis, have markedly improved image registration, target localization, image synthesis, and real-time image reconstruction in routine practice. This is particularly valuable as AI tools have enabled us to perform the tasks that cannot be accomplished using classical approaches, including real-time volumetric image reconstruction, image translation between MRI and CT. The additional gains will enable more accurate beam delivery, reduced toxicity, and improved treatment outcome.

References

[1] Jaffray D A 2012 Image-guided radiotherapy: from current concept to future perspectives *Nat. Rev. Clin. Oncol.* **9** 688–99

[2] Xing L *et al* 2006 Overview of image-guided radiation therapy *Med. Dosim.* **31** 91–112

[3] Barney B M *et al* 2011 Image-guided radiotherapy (IGRT) for prostate cancer comparing kV imaging of fiducial markers with cone beam computed tomography (CBCT) *Int. J. Radiat. Oncol. Biol. Phys.* **80** 301–5

[4] Western C, Hristov D and Schlosser J 2015 Ultrasound imaging in radiation therapy: from interfractional to intrafractional guidance *Cureus* **7** e280

[5] Price G J *et al* 2011 Real-time optical measurement of the dynamic body surface for use in guided radiotherapy *Phys. Med. Biol.* **57** 415

[6] Mutic S and Dempsey J F 2014 The ViewRay system: magnetic resonance–guided and controlled radiotherapy *Seminars in Radiation Oncology* (Amseterdam: Elsevier)

[7] Das S *et al* 2014 Comparison of image-guided radiotherapy technologies for prostate cancer *Am. J. Clin. Oncol.* **37** 616–23

[8] Shirato H *et al* 1999 Real-time tumour-tracking radiotherapy *Lancet* **353** 1331–2

[9] Freislederer P *et al* 2020 Recent advances in surface guided radiation therapy *Radiother. Oncol.* **15** 1–11

[10] Hoisak J D P *et al* 2020 *Surface Guided Radiation Therapy* (Boca Raton, FL: CRC Press)

[11] Batista V *et al* 2020 Clinical paradigms and challenges in surface guided radiation therapy: where do we go from here? *Radiother. Oncol.* **153** 34–42

[12] Bova F J *et al* 1997 The University of Florida frameless high-precision stereotactic radiotherapy system *Int. J. Radiat. Oncol. Biol. Phys.* **38** 875–82

[13] Lightstone A *et al* 2005 Intracranial stereotactic positioning systems: report of the American Association of Physicists in Medicine Radiation Therapy Committee task group no. 68 *Med. Phys.* **32** 2380–98

[14] Willoughby T *et al* 2012 Quality assurance for nonradiographic radiotherapy localization and positioning systems: report of Task Group 147 *Med. Phys.* **39** 1728–47

[15] Li R *et al* 2012 Evaluation of the geometric accuracy of surrogate-based gated VMAT using intrafraction kilovoltage x-ray images. *Med. Phys.* **39** 2686–93

[16] Rydhög J S *et al* 2017 Target position uncertainty during visually guided deep-inspiration breath-hold radiotherapy in locally advanced lung cancer *Radiother Oncol.* **123** 78–84

[17] Fassi A *et al* 2018 Target position reproducibility in left-breast irradiation with deep inspiration breath-hold using multiple optical surface control points. *J. Appl. Clin. Med. Phys.* **19** 35–43

[18] Vinogradskiy Y *et al* 2019 The clinical and dosimetric impact of real-time target tracking in pancreatic SBRT *Int. J. Radiat. Oncol. Biol. Phys.* **103** 268–75

[19] Hoisak J D and Pawlicki T 2018 The role of optical surface imaging systems in radiation therapy. in *Seminars in Radiation Oncology* (Amsterdam: Elsevier)

[20] Jaffray D A *et al* 2002 Flat-panel cone-beam computed tomography for image-guided radiation therapy *Int. J. Radiat. Oncol. Biol. Phys.* **53** 1337–49

[21] Jin J-Y *et al* 2008 Use of the brainLAB exactrac x-ray 6D system in image-guided radiotherapy *Med. Dosimet.* **33** 124–34

[22] Shirato H *et al* 2003 Feasibility of insertion/implantation of 2.0-mm-diameter gold internal fiducial markers for precise setup and real-time tumor tracking in radiotherapy *Int. J. Radiat. Oncol. Biol. Phys.* **56** 240–7

[23] Shirato H *et al* 2007 Organ motion in image-guided radiotherapy: lessons from real-time tumor-tracking radiotherapy *Int. J. Clin. Oncol.* **12** 8–16

[24] Fledelius W *et al* 2014 Real-time segmentation of multiple implanted cylindrical liver markers in kilovoltage and megavoltage x-ray images *Phys. Med. Biol.* **59** 2787

[25] Regmi R *et al* 2014 Automatic tracking of arbitrarily shaped implanted markers in kilovoltage projection images: a feasibility study *Med. Phys.* **41** 071906

[26] Kothary N *et al* 2009 Safety and efficacy of percutaneous fiducial marker implantation for image-guided radiation therapy *J. Vasc. Interv. Radiol.* **20** 235–9

[27] Adler J R Jr *et al* 1997 The Cyberknife: a frameless robotic system for radiosurgery *Stereotact. Funct. Neurosurg.* **69** 124–8

[28] Murphy M J *et al* 2000 Image-guided radiosurgery for the spine and pancreas *Comput. Aided Surg.* **5** 278–88

[29] Shirato H *et al* 2000 Physical aspects of a real-time tumor-tracking system for gated radiotherapy *Int. J. Radiat. Oncol. Biol. Phys.* **48** 1187–95

[30] Hashimoto T *et al* 2005 Real-time monitoring of a digestive tract marker to reduce adverse effects of moving organs at risk (OAR) in radiotherapy for thoracic and abdominal tumors *Int. J. Radiat. Oncol. Biol. Phys.* **61**(5) 1559–64

[31] Kinoshita R *et al* 2008 Three-dimensional intrafractional motion of breast during tangential breast irradiation monitored with high-sampling frequency using a real-time tumor-tracking radiotherapy system *Int. J. Radiat. Oncol. Biol. Phys.* **70** 931–34

[32] Paganelli C *et al* 2018 MRI-guidance for motion management in external beam radiotherapy: current status and future challenges *Phys. Med. Biol.* **63** 22TR03

[33] Raaymakers B W *et al* 2009 Integrating a 1.5 T MRI scanner with a 6 MV accelerator: proof of concept *Phys. Med. Biol.* **54** N229

[34] Glitzner M *et al* 2019 MLC-tracking performance on the elekta unity MRI-linac *Phys. Med. Biol.* **64** 15NT02

[35] Harris E, Fontanarosa D and Baldock C 2021 In the future, ultrasound guidance in radiotherapy will become a clinical standard *Phys. Eng. Sci. Med.* **44** 347–50

[36] Molloy J A *et al* 2011 Quality assurance of US-guided external beam radiotherapy for prostate cancer: report of AAPM Task Group 154. *Med. Phys.* **38** 857–71

[37] Lachaine M and Falco T 2013 Intrafractional prostate motion management with the Clarity Autoscan system *Med. Phys. Int.* **1** 72–80

[38] Grimwood A *et al* 2018 In vivo validation of Elekta's Clarity Autoscan for ultrasound-based intrafraction motion estimation of the prostate during radiation therapy *Int. J. Radiat. Oncol. Biol. Phys.* **102** 912–21

[39] Godfrey D J *et al* 2006 Digital tomosynthesis with an on-board kilovoltage imaging device *Int. J. Radiat. Oncol. Biol. Phys.* **65** 8–15

[40] Jiang Z *et al* 2021 Enhancing digital tomosynthesis (DTS) for lung radiotherapy guidance using patient-specific deep learning model *Phys. Med. Biol.* **66** 035009

[41] Pang G *et al* 2008 Megavoltage cone beam digital tomosynthesis (MV-CBDT) for image-guided radiotherapy: a clinical investigational system *Phys. Med. Biol.* **53** 999

[42] Yan H and Dai J-R 2017 Integrated digital tomosynthesis for patient positioning of image-guided radiation therapy *Physica Medica* **36** 24–31

[43] Hsieh S S and Ng L W 2017 Real-time tomosynthesis for radiation therapy guidance *Med. Phys.* **44** 5584–95

[44] Du M, Liu N and Hu X 2019 Techniques for interpretable machine learning *Commun. ACM* **63** 68–77

[45] Lin T *et al* 2009 Markerless gating for lung cancer radiotherapy based on machine learning techniques *Phys. Med. Biol.* **54** 1555

[46] Mylonas A *et al* 2019 A deep learning framework for automatic detection of arbitrarily shaped fiducial markers in intrafraction fluoroscopic images *Medical physics* **46** 2286–97

[47] Liao R *et al* 2017 An artificial agent for robust image registration *Proc. of the AAAI Conf. on Artificial Intelligence* 4168–75

[48] Fu Y *et al* 2020 LungRegNet: an unsupervised deformable image registration method for 4D-CT lung. *Med. Phys.* **47** 1763–74

[49] Zhao S *et al* 2019 Unsupervised 3D end-to-end medical image registration with volume tweening network *IEEE J. Biomed. Health Inform.* **24** 1394–404

[50] Jiang Z *et al* 2020 A multi-scale framework with unsupervised joint training of convolutional neural networks for pulmonary deformable image registration *Phys. Med. Biol.* **65** 015011

[51] Langen K M *et al* 2008 Observations on real-time prostate gland motion using electromagnetic tracking *Int. J. Radiat. Oncol. Biol. Phys.* **71** 1084–90

[52] van der Wielen G J *et al* 2008 Deformation of prostate and seminal vesicles relative to intraprostatic fiducial markers *Int. J. Radiat. Oncol. Biol. Phys.* **72** 1604–11. e3

[53] Gauthier I *et al* 2009 Dosimetric impact and theoretical clinical benefits of fiducial markers for dose escalated prostate cancer radiation treatment *Int. J. Radiat. Oncol. Biol. Phys.* **74** 1128–33

[54] Jayachandran P *et al* 2010 Interfractional uncertainty in the treatment of pancreatic cancer with radiation *Int. J. Radiat. Oncol. Biol. Phys.* **76** 603–7

[55] Sanders M K *et al* 2010 EUS-guided fiducial placement for stereotactic body radiotherapy in locally advanced and recurrent pancreatic cancer *Gastrointest. Endosc.* **71** 1178–84

[56] Gurney-Champion O J *et al* 2015 Visibility and artifacts of gold fiducial markers used for image guided radiation therapy of pancreatic cancer on MRI *Med. Phys.* **42** 2638–47

[57] Zhao W *et al* 2019 Incorporating imaging information from deep neural network layers into image guided radiation therapy (IGRT) *Radiother. Oncol.* **140** 167–74

[58] Zhao W *et al* 2019 Markerless pancreatic tumor target localization enabled by deep learning *Int. J. Radiat. Oncol. Biol. Phys.* **105** 432–39

[59] Zhao W *et al* 2018 Visualizing the invisible in prostate radiation therapy: markerless prostate target localization via a deep learning model and monoscopic kv projection x-ray image *Int. J. Radiat. Oncol. Biol. Phys.* **102** S128–9

[60] Zhao W *et al* 2019 Automatic marker-free target positioning and tracking for image-guided radiotherapy and interventions in medical imaging *Image-Guided Procedures, Robotic Interventions, and Modeling* (Bellingham, WA: SPIE)

[61] Zhao W *et al* 2019 Deep learning approach for markerless pancreatic tumor target localization *Int. J. Radiat. Oncol. Biol. Phys.* **105** S202–3

[62] Zhao W *et al* 2020 Fiducial-free image-guided spinal stereotactic radiosurgery enabled via deep learning *Int. J. Radiat. Oncol. Biol. Phys.* **108** e357

[63] Jaffray D A *et al* 2002 Flat-panel cone-beam computed tomography for image-guided radiation therapy *Int. J. Radiat. Oncol. Biol. Phys.* **53** 1337–49

[64] Oldham M *et al* 2005 Cone-beam-CT guided radiation therapy: a model for on-line application *Radiother. Oncol.* **75** 271

[65] Den R B *et al* 2010 Daily image guidance with cone-beam computed tomography for head-and-neck cancer intensity-modulated radiotherapy: a prospective study *Int. J. Radiat. Oncol. Biol. Phys.* **76** 1353–9
[66] Grills I S *et al* 2008 Image-guided radiotherapy via daily online cone-beam CT substantially reduces margin requirements for stereotactic lung radiotherapy *Int. J. Radiat. Oncol. Biol. Phys.* **70** 1045–56
[67] Shi W *et al* 2011 Evaluation of kV cone-beam CT performance for prostate IGRT: a comparison of automatic grey-value alignment to implanted fiducial-marker alignment *American J. Clinc. Oncol.* **34** 16–21
[68] Deegan T *et al* 2015 Assessment of cone beam CT registration for prostate radiation therapy: fiducial marker and soft tissue methods *J. Med. Imaging. Radiat. Oncol.* **59** 91–8
[69] Yildirim B A, Onal C and Dolek Y 2017 Is it essential to use fiducial markers during cone-beam CT-based radiotherapy for prostate cancer patients? *Jpn. J. Radiol.* **35** 3–9
[70] Kamino Y *et al* Development of a four-dimensional image-guided radiotherapy system with a gimbaled x-ray head 2006 *Int. J. Radiat. Oncol. Biol. Phys.* **66** 271–8
[71] Bertholet J *et al* 2018 Automatic online and real-time tumour motion monitoring during stereotactic liver treatments on a conventional linac by combined optical and sparse monoscopic imaging with kilovoltage x-rays (COSMIK) *Phys. Med. Biol.* **63** 055012
[72] Keall P J *et al* 2015 The first clinical treatment with kilovoltage intrafraction monitoring (KIM): a real-time image guidance method *Med. Phys.* **42** 354–8
[73] Willoughby T R *et al* 2006 Target localization and real-time tracking using the calypso 4D localization system in patients with localized prostate cancer *Int. J. Radiat. Oncol. Biol. Phys.* **65** 528–34
[74] Balter J M *et al* 2005 Accuracy of a wireless localization system for radiotherapy *Int. J. Radiat. Oncol. Biol. Phys.* **61** 933–7
[75] Hazelaar C *et al* 2018 First experience with markerless online 3D spine position monitoring during SBRT delivery using a conventional LINAC *Int. J. Radiat. Oncol. Biol. Phys.* **101** 1253–8
[76] Poulsen P R *et al* 2008 Three-dimensional prostate position estimation with a single x-ray imager utilizing the spatial probability density *Phys. Med. Biol.* **53** 4331
[77] Ng J A *et al* 2014 Quality assurance for the clinical implementation of kilovoltage intrafraction monitoring for prostate cancer VMAT *Med. Phys.* **41** 111712
[78] Poulsen P R *et al* 2014 Kilovoltage intrafraction motion monitoring and target dose reconstruction for stereotactic volumetric modulated arc therapy of tumors in the liver *Radiother. Oncol.* **111** 424–30
[79] Jones B L, Schefter T and Miften M 2015 Adaptive motion mapping in pancreatic SBRT patients using Fourier transforms *Radiother. Oncol.* **115** 217–22
[80] Ng J A *et al* 2012 Kilovoltage intrafraction monitoring for prostate intensity modulated arc therapy: first clinical results *Int. J. Radiat. Oncol. Biol. Phys.* **84** e655–61
[81] Keall P J *et al* 2016 Real-time 3D image guidance using a standard LINAC: measured motion, accuracy, and precision of the first prospective clinical trial of kilovoltage intra-fraction monitoring–guided gating for prostate cancer radiation therapy *Int. J. Radiat. Oncol. Biol. Phys.* **94** 1015–21
[82] Nguyen D T *et al* 2017 The first clinical implementation of a real-time six degree of freedom target tracking system during radiation therapy based on Kilovoltage Intrafraction Monitoring (KIM) *Radiother. Oncol.* **123** 37–42

[83] Kim J *et al* 2017 Quantifying the accuracy and precision of a novel real-time 6 degree-of-freedom kilovoltage intrafraction monitoring (KIM) target tracking system *Phys. Med. Biol.* **62** 5744

[84] Deutschmann H *et al* 2012 First clinical release of an online, adaptive, aperture-based image-guided radiotherapy strategy in intensity-modulated radiotherapy to correct for inter-and intrafractional rotations of the prostate *Int. J. Radiat. Oncol. Biol. Phys.* **83** 1624–32

[85] Poulsen P R *et al* 2012 Megavoltage image-based dynamic multileaf collimator tracking of a NiTi stent in porcine lungs on a linear accelerator *Int. J. Radiat. Oncol. Biol. Phys.* **82** e321–7

[86] Richter A *et al* 2010 Feasibility study for markerless tracking of lung tumors in stereotactic body radiotherapy *Int. J. Radiat. Oncol. Biol. Phys.* **78** 618–27

[87] Aristophanous M *et al* 2011 EPID-guided 3D dose verification of lung SBRT *Med. Phys.* **38** 495–503

[88] Rottmann J, Keall P and Berbeco R 2013 Markerless EPID image guided dynamic multi-leaf collimator tracking for lung tumors *Phys. Med. Biol.* **58** 4195

[89] Wan H, Ge J and Parikh P 2014 Using dynamic programming to improve fiducial marker localization *Phys. Med. Biol.* **59** 1935

[90] Li R *et al* 2010 Real-time volumetric image reconstruction and 3D tumor localization based on a single x-ray projection image for lung cancer radiotherapy *Med. Phys.* **37** 2822–6

[91] Li R *et al* 2011 3D tumor localization through real-time volumetric x-ray imaging for lung cancer radiotherapy *Med. Phys.* **38** 2783–94

[92] Shen L, Zhao W and Xing L 2019 Patient-specific reconstruction of volumetric computed tomography images from a single projection view via deep learning *Nat. Biomed. Eng.* **3** 880–8

[93] Tuy H K 1983 An inversion formula for cone-beam reconstruction *SIAM J. Appl. Math.* **43** 546–52

[94] Smith B D 1985 Image reconstruction from cone-beam projections: necessary and sufficient conditions and reconstruction methods *IEEE Trans. on Med. Imaging* **4** 14–25

[95] Lei Y *et al* 2020 Deep learning-based real-time volumetric imaging for lung stereotactic body radiation therapy: a proof of concept study *Phys. Med. Biol.* **65** 235003

Chapter 9

AI for quality management in radiation therapy

Quan Chen, Yi Rong, Zhichao Wang and Tianye Niu

Quality management consists of activities designed to ensure the desired quality and safety goals can be met. In terms of radiation therapy, these goals include, but are not limited to, accurate target and organ delineation, machine characterization, delivery of the planned dose distribution to the desired location, accurate dose recording and verification, etc. A radiation therapy treatment with insufficient quality control and management will inevitably lead to poor treatment outcomes, and even a risk to patient safety. While every member of the health care team is responsible for quality and safety, clinical medical physicists' duties and activities are more focused on this aspect, and thus carry greater responsibilities in terms of treatment accuracy. Recent advancement in artificial intelligence presents strong utility in quality management for medical physics and radiation therapy, which is the main focus of this chapter.

9.1 QA versus QC

Quality control (QC) and quality assurance (QA) are two important while distinct concepts in quality management (QM). In a general context, QA is defined as 'part of quality management that focuses on *providing confidence* that quality requirement will be fulfilled', while QC is defined as 'part of quality management that focused on *fulfilling* quality requirements'. Note that the roles of QC or QA for the same QM activities are interchangeable when viewed from a different perspective. An output from a process usually can become an input to the other. Thus, a QA for the first process may become a QC for the next. For example, a Linac output verification is a QA activity for the Linac tweaking and calibration process. At the same time, it serves as a QC step for ensuring precise treatment delivery. Because of these definition crossovers, the distinctions are often indistinct in radiation therapy practice and physicists often refer all their quality management activities as 'QA'.

Medical physicists perform various QM tasks to ensure quality and safety of the overall process of radiation therapy. The most important aspect is the establishment

doi:10.1088/978-0-7503-3339-9ch9

of a quality management program with consideration of the resources and clinical practices at their own facility. AAPM TG-100 [1] advocates for risk-based quality programs to enable each facility to direct resources most efficaciously towards patient safety and treatment quality as needed. These quality programs will include traditional QA/QC tasks, including chart reviews (initial check, weekly check, and close-out), machine QA (mechanical, dosimetric, imaging, safety interlocks, etc), treatment planning system QA, patient specific QA (including independent dose calculation, MU check, and delivery measurement), etc.

9.2 AI for chart review

Physics chart review is a review process of a patient's chart by physicists to help ensure quality and safety of a planned treatment. This activity is performed prior to the start of a patient's treatment (initial chart review), during the course of a treatment (weekly chart review) and at the completion of a treatment course (chart close-out review). In particular, the initial chart check has been identified as one of the most important QC checks. The reasons are two-fold. First, studies have shown that most errors in radiotherapy occur *before* the start of treatment [2, 3]. Second, studies comparing different QC checks show that the initial physics chart review is the most effective QC check for detecting severe errors [4]. Interestingly, weekly physics chart reviews were identified as the second most effective QC checks [4].

Despite high expectation in error detection during the initial chart reviews, near-misses or human errors can still slip through multiple layers of chart reviews in clinical practices. Gopan *et al* examined three years of potentially severe near-miss events from a single institution and found that 62% of the detectable errors had slipped through the initial chart review [5]. As chart reviews involve repetitive checks of plan parameters, it is highly likely that the human plan checker would be fatigued during the chart review process. It has been suggested that computer automation tools can improve the effectiveness and efficiency for most chart review checks [5]. Another advantage using automation is that it frees up physicists time so that they can focus their attention on other non-automated tasks that are also important for the safety and quality of patients' treatment.

Multiple tools have been developed to automate the chart review process. Due to the nature of the chart review process, most of those tools were implemented as an *expert system* where rules and logics used by a human plan checker were programmed as a knowledge base and inference engine respectively. An electronic radiation therapy plan quality assurance (QA) system (EQS) was developed at the University of Iowa [6] and later evolved into CATERS (computer aided treatment event recognition system) [7]. This system performs simple checks to ensure plan transfer integrity as well as various logic checks to detect inconsistencies such as planned dose mismatching with prescription. A similar tool was developed at University of Michigan [8] to automate part of the chart checking tasks. Researchers from Washington University in St. Louis also developed an automated chart check tool [9, 10] that has went through many rounds of improvements to add more capabilities, including the verification of treatment delivery with EPID [11] for weekly chart review, and adaptations to new treatment modalities [12–14]. In addition to the research groups named above, other researchers [15–17] as well as commercial vendors have also developed automated chart review tools, including ClearCheck/ChartCheck from Radformation Inc., Mobius3D/MobiusFX from Varian Medical Systems, and PlanCheck/PlanIQ from Sun Nuclear Corp.

While chart review expert systems have demonstrated their value in catching errors and saving human operation time, there are many limitations for wider adoption in clinical practice. One of the challenges is that there are a variety of treatment machines, treatment planning systems and oncology information systems (OIS) which produce many possible combinations across different clinics. In addition, clinical practices for the same disease may vary across institutions or even between oncologists in the same institution, including prescription, fractionation scheme, tolerance dose, naming conventions, etc. Clinical adoption of the chart review expert system developed at a different institution may require extensive changes to the knowledge base and inference engines. These changes, when not fully implemented and validated, will lead to undetected errors. Siochi *et al* evaluated error detection capabilities of their system and discovered that some errors were missed because the system mishandled the changes brought about by the implementation of new processes [6]. While there were efforts to improve its versality such as obtaining plan information from PDF parsing [18, 19], the chart review expert system remains rigid and requires high-maintenance.

With the success of big data and machine learning (ML) and deep learning (DL) in many fields, many research groups started to investigate the feasibility of using ML for automated chart review. The ML approach has the technical advantage of 'learning' how a specific institution operates without the need to modify the program. Early attempts involve detecting 'outliers' from all treatment plans. The advantage of this approach is that it doesn't need labeled data (cases that have known errors) as the errors are relatively infrequent and may slip through detection. One proof-of-concept study uses a *k*-means algorithm to detect outliers in historic 'four field' box treatment of prostate patients [20]. To demonstrate the robustness of the learning-based approach in handling data from different institutions, El Naqa *et al* developed a nonlinear kernel mapping with support vector data description (SVDD) driven approaches on data from eight Linacs in seven institutions, using portal imaging devices for catching gantry sag, radiation field shift, and MLC offset acquired using electronic portal imaging devices were analyzed for outliers [21].

The outlier classifiers mentioned above can produce a classification without explicit probability, which places higher requirement for tuning and enhancing performance of the classifier. Bayesian network processes a more explicit usage of probability and improves interpretability in application. Usually, an initial Bayesian network was constructed through expert knowledge, and machine learning methods were utilized to calculate a conditional probability table and update the network through treatment data. When checking a new treatment plan, a low probability in the network can corresponded to potential errors to be flagged for investigation. Kalet *et al* constructed a Bayesian network using the expectation maximization method [22]. The trained model, in error detection, performed as well as a domain expert in lung and breast. A Bayesian network topology, more complex than the previous paper, was constructed and different classes of errors were also introduced [23]. Results showed that classes of errors commonly encountered in radiotherapy planning could be detected. Since data collection was collected over ten years with continuous evolution in radiotherapy treatment plans, the authors also researched the optimal time period of data for the training of Bayesian networks [23]. Chang *et al* utilized three different Bayesian networks, trained with Bayesian learning algorithms, to detect errors in three different types of physician orders for external beam radiation therapy: single prescription, concurrent boost, and sequential boost [24]. Results reported reasonable true positive and false positive rates for different diseases.

AAPM TG-275 performed failure modes and effects analysis (FMEA) to rank the importance of errors that should be caught by physics chart review, among which 'wrong' or inaccurate contours ranked top [25]. Various methods were developed to automatically detect inaccurately drawn contours. A random forest model was built to learn joint distributions of contour features [26]. The trained model could automatically detect contour mislabeling errors, and it could also automatically assess the consistency of contour of segmentation on different CT slices. Chen *et al* applied geometric attribute distribution models with radiation therapy simulation images and contours of a given patient as input [27]. The results showed the trained model has high specificity and sensitivity. Hui *et al* used a statistical approach to detect inaccurate organs at risk (OAR) contours [28]. Various features for OAR were computed from training cases to construct a reference database. A multicriteria outlier detection system warns users of outliers based on combinations of deviant features [28]. It was found that the tool is capable of detecting 94% of the mimicked errors and it improved the error detection sensitivity of chart review process. Similar work was performed on the quality assurance of head and neck contours with encouraging results [29].

The use of AI for quality assurance and error detection is in two main categories: patient plan QA and dose delivery machine QA. AI for patient plan QA includes plan delivery accuracy, plan error detection, or plan checking process automation. AI for delivery machine QA includes output variation and dose profiles prediction, or machine mechanical error detection.

9.3 AI for patient specific QA and gamma passing rate prediction

Patient specific QA provides a phantom simulated end-to-end dose delivery verification to ensure no errors are made in the process of plan creation, TPS modeling, and file transfer. This time-consuming process has traditionally been performed manually by medical physicists for each patient plan. Recently, machine learning or deep learning AI has been investigated in this area to introduce automation or potential error prediction or detection. Valdes *et al* (2016) gathered 498 treatment plans and constructed a Poisson regression model with Lasso regularization to predict the gamma passing rate (GPR, 3%/3 mm local dose/distance-to-agreement (DTA)), with 78 metrics describing the complexity of treatment plans (input) [30]. Results showed that, for all plans analyzed, GPR prediction is accurate to within 3%. A weighted Poisson regression model with Lasso regularization was further studied for the same purpose, but with an independent dataset of 130 plans from another institution, using 90 metrics describing complexity of treatment plans as input and the same GPR index as output [31]. Low prediction errors were observed for both institutions, showing a potential of generalizing the same model for different institutions when certain IMRT QA parameters are unified. This study did not address the prediction for plan QA results in terms of pass or fail. Li *et al* trained two models with 54 metrics as input: Poisson lasso regression to predict gamma passing rate at 3%/3 mm, 3%/2 mm and 2%/2 mm criterion, and random forest regression to predict QA pass/fail result [32]. Poisson lasso regression was shown a higher specificity (identifying plans that can pass QA), whereas random forest regression a higher sensitivity (identifying plans that cannot pass QA). Ono *et al* applied three different models: regression tree analysis, multiple regression analysis and neural network to build the relationship between input features and output GPR [33]. In terms of accuracy of GPR prediction, neural network performed slightly better than regression tree analysis, multiple regression analysis. Lam *et al* also constructed three different tree-based models: AdaBoost, random forest, and XGBoost [34]. All of these methods predicted GPR accurately, although XGBoost worked slightly less well than the other two methods. Quite differently, Wall *et al* obtained input features using forests of extra-trees, mutual information, and linear regression [35]. Multiple models including linear models, support vector machines, tree-based models, and neural networks were applied, and support vector machine had the best performance. None of the above mentioned papers considered dosimetric aspects of the IMRT QA. To improve the performance of the machine learning model, dosimetric features were added as input to train XGBoost model, and significant improvement in GPR prediction was observed [36]. Granville *et al* utilized linear support vector classifier to classify the difference between planned and delivered dose distribution as 'hot', 'normal' and 'cold' [37]. The input to the model included features describing treatment plan complexity and linac performance, while the output was median dose deviation. This paper showed potential of using both treatment plan characteristics and routine linac QC results to realize QA of treatment delivery.

The literature also presents deep learning convolutional neural networks (CNN) for GPR prediction of patient plan QA. Tomori *et al* proposed building a fifteen-layer CNN to predict GPR with volume of the PTV and OAR and the monitor unit values in each field as input [38]. A strong correlation was discovered between predicted and measured GPR. Another CNN inspired by VGG-16 was constructed and trained through transfer learning with fluence map extracted from treatment plan as input [39]. Comparison with the machine learning method, where input metrics were designed by experts, the performance of CNN was comparable. Brown *et al* combined five widely used imbalanced-data classification with filtering methods for imbalanced data [40]. The authors discovered that the trained model had strong performance in identifying unacceptable treatment plans.

9.4 AI for dosimetric and mechanical QA for linear accelerators

A medical linear accelerator (linac) is commonly used for external beam radiation treatments for cancer patients. Linac requires multi-layers of machine QA at various frequencies, including daily, weekly, monthly, and annual. These QA procedures ensure accurate delivery of x-ray to tumor target, while those adjacent organs at risk are spared. Valdes *et al* proposed using a support vector machine to accomplish daily imaging QA and monthly imaging QA tests for SRS and SBRT protocols [41]. The input to the model was cone beam CT (CBCT), and the model could identify and remove artifacts. This automation has two strengths: reduced time for the QA process and successful identification of most kinds of artifacts. In similar research, artificial neural networks (ANNs) and autoregressive moving average (ARMA) models were constructed based on five year daily linac QA data [42]. Results showed that ANN was superior to ARMA for QA.

9.4.1 Output factor and monitor unit

For proton therapy, one of the challenges is to convert the prescribed dose to the machine deliverable monitor units (MU). Output factor (OF), i.e., dose per MU (d/MU), played the role of an intermediary between dose and MU. In reality, OF was determined with measurements prior to treatment, and it was quite time consuming. To facilitate the process of obtaining OF, several research papers have been published about prediction OF using machine learning and deep learning models.

Different machine learning models, including random forest, XGBoost and cubist, were constructed to predict output factors and further derive MUs, with option number, range, and modulation width as input [43]. The results showed that cubist outperformed other methods, and all of these machine learning methods were superior to traditional semi-empirical methods. Grewal *et al* applied both Gaussian process regression and shallow neural network to predict OF [44]. In the training process, range, modulation, field size, and measured output factor were included as input, while only the first three parameters were utilized for the test process. The prediction accuracy of machine and deep learning algorithms is higher than the empirical method.

9.4.2 Linac mechanical error detection

Multileaf collimator (MLC) is an important part in the dose delivery pathway that requires sufficient quality control. The main research work focuses on MLC error detection and classification. Wootton *et al* utilized logistic regression with radiomic features extracted from a gamma image as input and the output was the likelihood of error [45]. It was demonstrated that the model performed better than traditional threshold-based gamma analysis in error detection, and it could also discriminate the two errors. To accomplish a similar goal, Nyflot *et al* constructed four machine learning classifiers: support vector machines, multilayer perceptrons, decision trees, and k-nearest-neighbors, to detect errors with extracted features as input [46]. Two classification problems were included in the process: classification 1: error free or containing MLC error; classification 2: error free, containing MLC systemic error or containing MLC random error. The extracted features were obtained either from CNN with triplet learning or handcrafted. The result showed that the deep learning approach was superior to the handcrafted feature selection approach and threshold-based passing criteria. Previous work on MLC error detection and classification was limited to IMRT, Kimura *et al* expanded Nyflot's work to VMAT [47]. In Kimura's CNN, the input was dose difference maps, and the output was the probability for error free, MLC systemic errors, and MLC random errors (the summation of these three is unity). The use of a dose difference map as input could obtain more accurate error prediction, compared to the study using gamma maps (Nyflot *et al*) [46, 47].

There are also publications on estimation of difference between the planned and delivered MLC positions. Several machine learning models, including linear regression, random forest, and cubist were constructed to predict the differences between the planned and delivered MLC positions with the leaf motion parameters as inputs [48]. The data were from three different institutions, and as a result, the training dataset contained three treatment plans (each one from a different institute) while the test set contained two treatment plans from two different institutions. The cubist model outperformed other methods, and the final model was capable of predicting MLC positions during delivery to a high degree of accuracy. Different from the previous work, Osman *et al* constructed an artificial neural network with 14 parameters extracted from log files as input and MLC leaf positional deviations as output [49]. The proposed artificial neural network was capable of accurately predicting the individual MLC leaf positional deviations during the dynamic IMRT delivery.

9.5 Summary

Overall, the literature has shown promising results in applying machine learning and deep learning models for computer automated error detection in QA and QM aspects in radiation therapy. Even though very few studies have been widely adopted for clinical uses yet, the entire field is heading in the direction of having more artificial intelligence and computer automation, thus reducing any severe consequences from human errors or negligence. Limitations still exist in various aspects, including high demand for good quality training datasets for AI and ML based model building, difficulties in model generalization and adaptation, inconsistency in detection accuracy and specificity, etc. Moreover, there may be a large portion of tests and tasks that can never be replaced by computer automation. Human intervention is still a crucial part of the entire QA and QC process for radiation oncology quality management.

References

[1] Huq M S *et al* 2016 The report of task group 100 of the AAPM: application of risk analysis methods to radiation therapy quality management *Med. Phys.* **43** 4209

[2] Clark B G *et al* 2010 The management of radiation treatment error through incident learning *Radiother. Oncol.* **95** 344–9

[3] Novak A *et al* 2016 Targeting safety improvements through identification of incident origination and detection in a near-miss incident learning system *Med. Phys.* **43** 2053–62
[4] Ford E C *et al* 2012 Quality control quantification (QCQ): a tool to measure the value of quality control checks in radiation oncology *Int. J. Radiat. Oncol. Biol. Phys.* **84** e263–9
[5] Gopan O *et al* 2016 The effectiveness of pretreatment physics plan review for detecting errors in radiation therapy *Med. Phys.* **43** 5181
[6] Siochi R A *et al* 2009 Radiation therapy plan checks in a paperless clinic *J. Appl. Clin. Med. Phys.* **10** 2905
[7] Xia J, Mart C and Bayouth J 2014 A computer aided treatment event recognition system in radiation therapy *Med. Phys.* **41** 011713
[8] Covington E L *et al* 2016 Improving treatment plan evaluation with automation *J. Appl. Clin. Med. Phys.* **17** 16–31
[9] Yang D and Moore K L 2012 Automated radiotherapy treatment plan integrity verification *Med. Phys.* **39** 1542–51
[10] Yang D *et al* 2012 Technical note: electronic chart checks in a paperless radiation therapy clinic *Med. Phys.* **39** 4726–32
[11] Liu S *et al* 2017 A method to reconstruct and apply 3D primary fluence for treatment delivery verification *J. Appl. Clin. Med. Phys.* **18** 128–38
[12] Cai B *et al* 2018 A practical implementation of physics quality assurance for photon adaptive radiotherapy *Z. Med. Phys.* **28** 211–23
[13] Sun B *et al* 2018 A machine learning approach to the accurate prediction of monitor units for a compact proton machine *Med. Phys.* **45** 2243–51
[14] Yang D *et al* 2016 A software tool to automatically assure and report daily treatment deliveries by a cobalt-60 radiation therapy device *J. Appl. Clin. Med. Phys.* **17** 492–501
[15] Furhang E E *et al* 2009 Automating the initial physics chart checking process *J. Appl. Clin. Med. Phys.* **10** 129–35
[16] Dewhurst J M *et al* 2015 AutoLock: a semiautomated system for radiotherapy treatment plan quality control *J. Appl. Clin. Med. Phys.* **16** 5396
[17] Olsen L A *et al* 2014 Automated radiation therapy treatment plan workflow using a commercial application programming interface *Pract. Radiat. Oncol.* **4** 358–67
[18] Halabi T and Lu H M 2014 Automating checks of plan check automation *J. Appl. Clin. Med. Phys.* **15** 4889
[19] Halabi T *et al* 2016 Automated survey of 8000 plan checks at eight facilities *Med. Phys.* **43** 4966
[20] Azmandian F *et al* 2007 Towards the development of an error checker for radiotherapy treatment plans: a preliminary study *Phys. Med. Biol.* **52** 6511–24
[21] El Naqa I *et al* 2019 Machine learning for automated quality assurance in radiotherapy: a proof of principle using EPID data description *Med. Phys.* **46** 1914–21
[22] Kalet A M *et al* 2015 Bayesian network models for error detection in radiotherapy plans *Phys. Med. Biol.* **60** 2735–49
[23] Luk S M H *et al* 2019 Characterization of a Bayesian network-based radiotherapy plan verification model *Med. Phys.* **46** 2006–14
[24] Chang X *et al* 2019 Development and validation of a Bayesian network method to detect external beam radiation therapy physician order errors *Int. J. Radiat. Oncol. Biol. Phys.* **105** 423–31
[25] Ford E *et al* 2020 Strategies for effective physics plan and chart review in radiation therapy: report of AAPM task group 275 *Med. Phys.* **47** e236–72

[26] McIntosh C, Svistoun I and Purdie T G 2013 Groupwise conditional random forests for automatic shape classification and contour quality assessment in radiotherapy planning *IEEE Trans. Med. Imaging* **32** 1043–57

[27] Chen H-C *et al* 2015 Automated contouring error detection based on supervised geometric attribute distribution models for radiation therapy: a general strategy *Med. Phys.* **42** 1048–59

[28] Hui C B *et al* 2018 Quality assurance tool for organ at risk delineation in radiation therapy using a parametric statistical approach *Med. Phys.* **45** 2089–96

[29] Altman M B *et al* 2015 A framework for automated contour quality assurance in radiation therapy including adaptive techniques *Phys. Med. Biol.* **60** 5199–209

[30] Valdes G *et al* 2016 A mathematical framework for virtual IMRT QA using machine learning *Med. Phys.* **43** 4323–34

[31] Valdes G *et al* 2017 IMRT QA using machine learning: a multi-institutional validation *J. Appl. Clin. Med. Phys.* **18** 279–84

[32] Li J *et al* 2019 Machine learning for patient-specific quality assurance of VMAT: prediction and classification accuracy *Int. J. Radiat. Oncol. Biol. Phys.* **105** 893–902

[33] Ono T *et al* 2019 Prediction of dosimetric accuracy for VMAT plans using plan complexity parameters via machine learning *Med. Phys.* **46** 3823–32

[34] Lam D *et al* 2019 Predicting gamma passing rates for portal dosimetry-based IMRT QA using machine learning *Med. Phys.* **46** 4666–75

[35] Wall P D H and Fontenot J D 2020 Application and comparison of machine learning models for predicting quality assurance outcomes in radiation therapy treatment planning *Inform. Med. Unlocked* **18** 100292

[36] Hirashima H *et al* 2020 Improvement of prediction and classification performance for gamma passing rate by using plan complexity and dosiomics features *Radiother. Oncol.* **153** 250–7

[37] Granville D A *et al* 2019 Predicting VMAT patient-specific QA results using a support vector classifier trained on treatment plan characteristics and linac QC metrics *Phys. Med. Biol.* **64** 095017

[38] Tomori S *et al* 2018 A deep learning-based prediction model for gamma evaluation in patient-specific quality assurance *Med. Phys.* **45** 4055–65

[39] Interian Y *et al* 2018 Deep nets vs expert designed features in medical physics: an IMRT QA case study *Med. Phys.* **45** 2672–80

[40] Brown W E *et al* 2018 Guided undersampling classification for automated radiation therapy quality assurance of prostate cancer treatment *Med. Phys.* **45** 1306–16

[41] Valdes G *et al* 2015 Use of truebeam developer mode for imaging QA *J. Appl. Clin. Med. Phys.* **16** 322–33

[42] Li Q and Chan M F 2017 Predictive time-series modeling using artificial neural networks for linac beam symmetry: an empirical study *Ann. N.Y. Acad. Sci.* **1387** 84–94

[43] Sun B *et al* 2018 A machine learning approach to the accurate prediction of monitor units for a compact proton machine *Med. Phys.* **45** 2243–51

[44] Grewal H S *et al* 2020 Prediction of the output factor using machine and deep learning approach in uniform scanning proton therapy *J. Appl. Clin. Med. Phys.* **21** 128–34

[45] Wootton L S *et al* 2018 Error detection in intensity-modulated radiation therapy quality assurance using radiomic analysis of gamma distributions *Int. J. Radiat. Oncol. Biol. Phys.* **102** 219–28

[46] Nyflot M J *et al* 2019 Deep learning for patient-specific quality assurance: Identifying errors in radiotherapy delivery by radiomic analysis of gamma images with convolutional neural networks *Med. Phys.* **46** 456–64

[47] Kimura Y *et al* 2020 Error detection using a convolutional neural network with dose difference maps in patient-specific quality assurance for volumetric modulated arc therapy *Phys. Med.* **73** 57–64

[48] Carlson J N K *et al* 2016 A machine learning approach to the accurate prediction of multi-leaf collimator positional errors *Phys. Med. Biol.* **61** 2514–31

[49] Osman A F I, Maalej N M and Jayesh K 2020 Prediction of the individual multileaf collimator positional deviations during dynamic IMRT delivery priori with artificial neural network *Med. Phys.* **47** 1421–30

Chapter 10

Data-driven approaches in radiotherapy outcome modeling

Ibrahim Chamseddine, Yejin Kim and Clemens Grassberger

Radiotherapy is one of the most quantitative disciplines within medicine, with a long tradition of outcome modeling and prediction. Traditional approaches in dose-outcome modeling have been limited by the heterogeneity among patients. This chapter will introduce the approaches that have been proposed to overcome this limitation, together with examples from radiation oncology. The purpose is to give both the medical physicist an insight into ML-based outcome modeling, as well as the machine learning expert an overview over the existing models and assumptions in radiation oncology that are often implicitly included in the data.

10.1 Introduction

What primarily differentiates outcome modeling in radiotherapy from other disciplines is the dose distribution as an important predictor of outcome. Radiotherapy outcome modeling has a long tradition, and early efforts to capture radiation-induced toxicities or to model local control consisted primarily of correlations of dose or dose-volume with effect. The focus has historically been on population-averaged constraints to keep the incidence of side effects below a certain level, and individualized predictions were impeded by the enormous heterogeneity among patients. Not only is cancer one of the most diverse and adaptable human diseases, making its response to therapy variable, the individual patient's normal tissue response to radiation is heterogenous as well.

Two current have emerged to address this issue: either integrate patient-specific factors into traditional outcome models, or to forfeit all structure and include dose via various mechanisms into purely data-driven approaches. This chapter gives an overview of both aspects and describes the elements of model building with a focus on radiotherapy outcome prediction and reference to specific applications.

doi:10.1088/978-0-7503-3339-9ch10

10.2 Analytical dose–response models and extensions

The classical models and concepts described here are unique to radiotherapy, and are often still included inherently in machine learning models, e.g., when dose is corrected beforehand to account for fractionation. They have also been extended into more data-driven approaches using variables other than dose, as described in the last section.

10.2.1 Linear-quadratic model and equivalent dose

The foundation of the linear-quadratic (LQ) model lies in basic radiation biology, as it is the common formalism to describe the clonogenic survival of cells *in vitro* after irradiation. In its most basic formation, the surviving fraction (SF) of cells after a radiation dose d is described by

$$\mathrm{SF} = e^{-(\alpha d+\beta d^2)} \tag{10.1}$$

where α and β are cell-type specific parameters that are fitted to experimental cell survival data [4]. This simple notation assumes delivery of dose at usual dose rates, for very low dose rates a protraction factor is be added to the quadratic term to include the effect of repair [5]. This simple model is enduring in outcome modeling as it is used for calculating iso-effective doses between different fractionation regimen and time courses. Dose distributions in patients, specifically in normal tissue, contain high- as well as low-dose regions that are irradiated with different fraction sizes leading to a varying biological effect. Therefore dose distributions are often normalized to the equivalent dose in 2 Gy fractions (EQD2). A total physical dose D given in n fractions of dose d, i.e., $D = nd$, is normalized to the dose that would have given an equal effect when given in 2 Gy fractions:

$$\mathrm{EQD2} = D\,\frac{d + \alpha/\beta}{2 + \alpha/\beta} \tag{10.2}$$

While this is intimately connected to the concept of biologically equivalent dose (BED) [6], which is used less frequently in outcome modeling, the two should not be confused [7]. In this 'biological effect' normalization of the physical dose, the α/β ratio of a tissue describes the fractionation sensitivity [8] and becomes the defining variable. This variable should be carefully selected based on the tissue and endpoint [9], and particularly for tumors the assumptions have changed over the past decade. While traditionally tumors were modeled using a high α/β ratio, multiple studies have shown significant heterogeneity among tumor types and particularly lower values for breast and prostate cancer [10]. For a modern overview and interpretation of LQ and BED modeling we refer to McMahon *et al* [4].

Large fraction sizes. It is well known that at larger doses per fraction, experimentally observed cell survival rates are significantly higher than linear-quadratic model predictions following a continuously bending survival curve [11]. Other approaches have been proposed to include these observations, such as the linear-quadratic-linear [12] and the universal survival curve models [13]. While they have improved fit to *in vitro* experiments, it has been shown that these models do not add predictive power when applied for studies describing clinical results [14, 17], and most modern studies use the LQ model also to convert between hypo-fractionated schedules [18, 19].

10.2.2 Tumor control probability and normal tissue complication probability

Tumor control probability (TCP) models describe the probability to locally control a tumor after irradiation to a specific *homogeneous* dose. The 'target-cell hypothesis' [20] assumed that all clonogenic cells need to be inactivated, and the ensuing models were built on the foundation of Poisson statistics [21]. Even though these models have a strong connection to the biological parameters and a mechanistic interpretation, they do not take heterogeneity within the tumor into account [22].

Logistic dose–response models are used more frequently, providing a pragmatic description of tumor control as a function of dose that is needed to control 50% of tumors (D_{50}) and a steepness parameter k

$$\mathrm{TCP}(d) = \frac{1}{1 + \exp\left(\frac{D_{50} - d}{k}\right)} \tag{10.3}$$

The situation in normal tissue is more complex, as normal organs are usually irradiated with non-uniform dose distributions. Therefore, we need a formalism to take different inhomogeneous dose distributions into account to predict normal tissue complication probability (NTCP). The most popular of these is the Lyman–Kutcher–Burman model (LKB), describing the sigmoidal dose–response curve of normal tissues with the following probit form:

$$\mathrm{NTCP} = \Phi\left(\frac{\mathrm{gEUD} - D_{50}}{m \cdot D_{50}}\right) \tag{10.4}$$

where $\Phi(x)$ is a probit function

$$\Phi(x) = \frac{1}{\sqrt{2\pi}} \int_{-\infty}^{x} \exp\left(\frac{-t^2}{2}\right) \mathrm{dt} = \frac{1}{2}\left[1 + \mathrm{erf}\left(\frac{x}{\sqrt{2}}\right)\right] \tag{10.5}$$

with $x = (\mathrm{gEUD} - D_{50})/(m \bullet D_{50})$ as in equation (10.4). The generalized equivalent uniform dose (gEUD) represents the dose which, if delivered uniformly to the entire organ, would produce the same radiobiological effect as the given heterogeneous dose distribution, as specified by the dose-volume histogram (DVH). The gEUD is calculated from the differential DVH pairs $\{D_i, v_i\}$ as:

$$g\mathrm{EUD} = \left(\sum i v_i D_i^{a}\right)^{1/a}, \; g\mathrm{EUD} \rightarrow \begin{matrix} D_{\min}, & a \rightarrow -\infty \\ D_{\mathrm{mean}}, & a = 1 \\ D_{\max}, & a \rightarrow \infty \end{matrix} \tag{10.6}$$

Instead of gEUD, LKB models often use similar DVH-reduction models such as effective dose (D_{eff}) or effective volume (V_{eff}) formulations [23, 24], which all have the purpose to weigh the importance of the varying dose levels given to different volumes of the organ into one equivalent value. gEUD can also be used for TCP calculations if inhomogenous doses are given to the tumor, using a negative *a* parameter to penalize cold spots.

The LKB model with gEUD (or D_{eff}/V_{eff}) has three parameters: a volume effect parameter to account for differences in tissue architecture, with $a = 1$ representing mean dose and $a > 1$ or $a < 1$ increasing the weight of the high- or low-dose regions respectively; the slope of the dose–response curve m; and the dose corresponding to a 50% complication probability D_{50}.

What is often overlooked is that in the entire modeling process there is an additional parameter—the α/β ratio that has been used beforehand to normalize the dose distribution to equivalent fraction sizes. This pre-processing also leads to a different scaling of high- and low-dose regions, similar to the volume effect parameter in the LKB model. Therefore it is important to use similar α/β ratios as comparable studies, otherwise the estimates of volume effect cannot be compared easily.

The models described above have been fitted exhaustively to clinical data, with the most comprehensive efforts for normal tissues being led by QUANTEC (quantitative analysis of normal tissue effects in the clinic) [25, 26]. As most of the data included in the QUANTEC reports were focused on conventionally fractionated studies in adults, the ensuing HyTEC [27] and PENTEC [28] efforts focused on stereotactic radiation therapy and pediatric populations, respectively. An excellent primer for modeling dose–response relationships using these traditional models has recently been published [29].

10.3 Overview of machine learning models

Machine learning (ML) models are synthesized directly from data without relying on physical and biological mechanisms. They extract patterns directly from clinical data to map patient-specific factors and treatment characteristics to outcome. They can consider mixed types of variables such as binary clinical characteristics, categorical or ordinal scales and continuous dose levels, and model dose–response relationships based on patient characteristics using advanced architectures. ML is used in radiotherapy usually to predict the occurrence of an event at a specific time (endpoint prediction), or the time elapsed before an event occurs (survival analysis).

Outcomes are measured by endpoints indicating treatment failure or toxicity. Death and recurrence are two types of treatment failure commonly considered in predictive modeling, either predicted using a time-dependent probability function or binary occurrences at a specific timepoint, e.g., one year survival. Toxicity endpoints are site-specific and usually binarized for simplicity, even when the underlying value is on a continuous or ordinal scale [30, 31].

10.3.1 Endpoint prediction: regression and classification

RT outcome prediction uses primarily supervised machine learning. *Regression* models predict a continuous outcome such as the probability of death, reduction in tumor size, and changes in blood biomarkers. *Classification* models on the other hand predict binary outcomes such as whether recurrence, death, and radiation-induced diseases occur or not. Indeed, classifiers are not limited to binary outcomes and can predict categorical output with multiple levels such as predicting a disease stage or organ performance score after radiation therapy. Multiple endpoints can also be predicted simultaneously, in which case a modification of the receiver-operating characteristic curve has to be employed to take into account multiple outcomes [32]. Such an approach has been used in multi-objective Bayesian networks for the joint prediction of tumor control and radiation toxicity in lung cancer [33].

Although regression and classification are usually described separately in the literature, they share common learning algorithms. Learning algorithm refers to the method of learning the data and extracting patterns from it. The evaluation of performance, however, significantly differs between regression and classification. We will describe the learning algorithms and examples for both models in this section and then discuss their evaluation criteria later in this section.

In the simplest form, the outcome (y) can be calculated as the weighted sum of the variables (x)

$$y = \beta_0 + \sum \beta_i x_i + e$$

The coefficients β_i measure the contribution of each variable to the outcome; β_0 is the value of the outcome when all the variables are zero; and e is the error term. This type of models is linear. Although it is easy to interpret, it ignores interaction between the variables. The classification counterpart of linear regression is the logistic regression, which models a binary outcome using a sigmoidal transformation of this additive model [34].

Linear models can fail when there is strong interaction between variables, but can be extended using interaction terms. Nonlinear models on the other hand follow an algorithmic path to treat complex interactions between predictors. Table 10.1 presents a non-exhaustive but practical overview of the major learning algorithms used in radiotherapy outcome prediction. The reader is referred to chapter 1 for a more detailed explanation of each method as well as other learning algorithms.

For models not including imaging data, logistic regression (or Cox regression for survival data, see section below), regularized or with preceding feature selection, often performs surprisingly well and should be used as a benchmark. Comparative studies show that when comparing classifiers, no single algorithm performs better across multiple datasets even for similar prediction problems [35].

Advanced neural network architectures are being used increasingly also without imaging data, often as an alternative to conventional feature selection in high-dimensional space. Particularly variational autoencoders, an unsupervised technique to learn latent representation, has been used to constrain large numbers of biomarkers (single nucleotide polymorphisms, cytokines, and micro-RNA) in the prediction of radiation pneumonitis [36]. The value of this technique has also been demonstrated outside of radiotherapy for pan-cancer data [37], and it could become an avenue to include high-dimensional omics data into RT outcome prediction.

Table 10.1. Overview of major learning algorithms used in outcome prediction, recommendations for their use, and major considerations to avoid model under- or overfitting.

Learning Algorithm	Representation
Linear algorithms: the outcome is the sum of independent variables. The model is easy to interpret but it ignores interactions between variables. **Linear regression** is used for regression **Logistic regression** is used for classification **Recommended use:** easy interpretation of results; variables do not interact	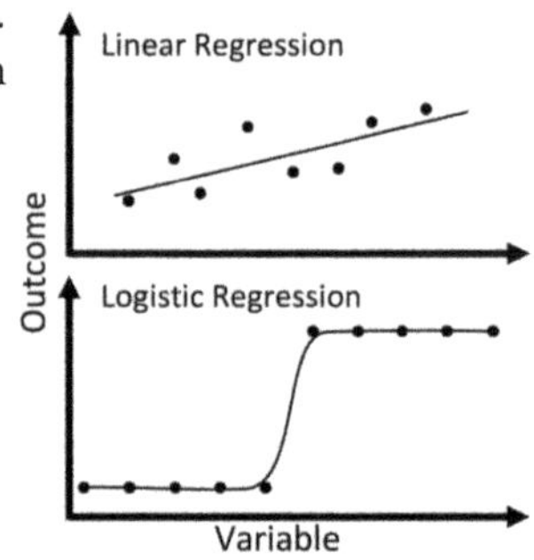
Separation algorithms: separate independent variables by class **Support vector machine** finds a hyperplane (decision boundary) that separates the variables with maximum margin **Recommended use:** nonlinear classification problems with binary outcome **Design considerations:** soft margins; maximum margin—distance between decision boundary and classes	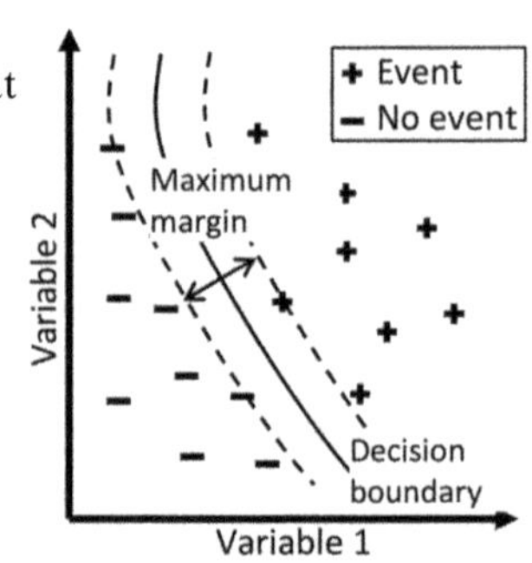
Tree-based algorithms: **Decision tree** consists of branches and nodes. Each node has a variable and a threshold for bifurcating the branch **Random forest** is an ensemble of trees trained independently on random subsets of data and/or features **Gradient boosted trees** is an ensemble of trees sequentially trained to reduce the error of previous trees **Recommended use:** many categorical or ordinal variables; many missing variables; nonlinear relationships **Design considerations:** number of trees, depth of trees, learning rate (in boosted trees)	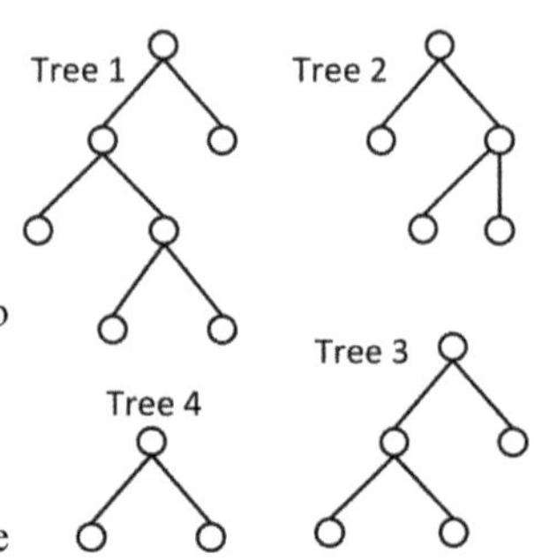
Neural networks: extract multilayer features from variables **Multilayer perceptron (MLP).** A perceptron is a linear classifier, a neural network composed of multiple layers of neurons and threshold activations. The fully connectedness of MLPs accounts for strong interactions among variables.	

Recommended use: both regression and classification; large numbers of variables; strong interaction between variables; extraction of multilayer features and feature engineering;
Design considerations: number of hidden layers; number of nodes in hidden layers; learning rate, dropout

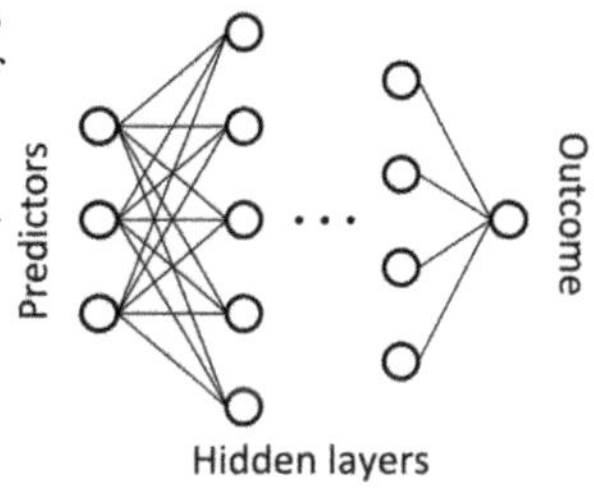

Long short-term memory networks, a recurrent neural network architecture popular for speech recognition and time-series data, can be used to include DVH data [30]. This incorporates the fact that DVH datapoints are not independent and will be discussed in more detail in section 10.4 focusing on including dosimetric information into outcome models.

In the case of high variability in the data, it is advisable to create multiple models and combine them in an *ensemble* of models [38]. Each model in an ensemble is trained on a resampled subset of the training dataset (see section 10.4 for different resampling procedures). All models then vote or are combined using a weighted average to predict the overall outcome. Alternatively, model *stacking* uses a meta-learner that tries to learn which models are reliable in which situations. This is often used when combining wildly different classifiers that perform well in different parts of feature space. Thor *et al* successfully used an ensemble of models aggregated by bootstrapping to improve their survival prediction after RT for lung cancer [39].

10.3.2 Inclusion of imaging data

Medical images are a rich source of information and widely used for outcome prediction outside of radiotherapy. Fundamentally, the integration of imaging data in RT outcome modeling is not different from other disciplines such as radiology or general oncology, and features two main approaches—*radiomics* [40] and *deep learning* [41]. Radiomics uses extraction of first and higher order statistical features from radiological images, while deep learning does not require engineered features as input for the framework. Given the high collinearity of radiomic features, proper feature selection and model building is critical (see section 10.4). A combination of radiomics with deep features from convolutional neural networks is gaining popularity, often termed transfer learning radiomics [42, 43].

Radiotherapy-specific applications of radiomics are emerging in differentiating tumor recurrence from other radiation-induced changes. In the brain radiomics features are both able to differentiate radionecrosis from progression after RT [44, 45], and predict response of brain necrosis after radiotherapy to bevacizumab [46]. Similarly, radiomics has been used after radiotherapy for lung cancer to distinguish local recurrence from the commonly occurring radiation-induced fibrosis [47]. Deep learning has been extensively applied to the assessment of response for bladder [48], pancreatic [49] and lung cancer patients after radiotherapy [50], and been extended using recurrent neural network structures that can take into account imaging at multiple timepoints [51]. As its application is often not specific to radiotherapy, we refer to the literature for details and applications of radiomics [40, 52] and deep learning [41, 53].

10.3.3 Survival prediction models

Survival analysis or time-to-event models describe the effect of variables on the time that passes before an event occurs. Although the term 'survival' is used, such models can be used for other types of events such as recurrence and toxicity. Survival prediction models can be thought of as a regression model for predicting the expected time to an event. The difference is that the time—which is the outcome here—is often *censored* [54]. In survival analysis data is usually right censored, meaning that the outcome in question has not occurred at the last time of observation. Another distinction from regression is that survival prediction models produce, rather than a predicted time to event, a survival function $S(t)$ that predicts the probability that the event has occurred at a time t for a subject with the given predictor variables ($P(T>t) = S(t)$). The shape of $S(t)$ and the coefficients for the predictors are estimated from a given set of survival data, in which information from censored subjects contributes to the model.

The most popular form of these models is the Cox regression model, which assumes that the hazard ratio is constant (proportional hazards assumption) and accounts for additive effects of covariates through exponential terms [39, 55]. Nonlinear algorithms can also be used to treat complex interactions between variables, most commonly random survival forests [56, 57].

10.3.4 Performance evaluation metrics

We mentioned earlier that regression and classification models share similar learning algorithms but have different evaluation criteria. In regression, the score focuses on the difference between the true and predicted value. Classification models in contrast are scored based on the number of correct and incorrect labeling of the data. Table 10.2 lists the common metrics used for scoring predictive models along with practical recommendations.

It is essential, particularly with complex models that use imaging data combined with clinical features, to compare model performance to simple models based only on clinical predictors [51]. Cui *et al* evaluated the combination of traditional machine learning methods for feature selection with deep learning techniques, and demonstrated significant improvement in AUC using the DeLong test from *U*-statistics. However, analysis of performance improvements should be undertaken with care, as the behavior of nested models often does not comply with the requirements of the statistical method used [58, 59].

When evaluating models that predict risk groups in patients subject to censoring, a more interpretable alternative to the c-indices is to use the Kaplan–Meier method and the log-rank test to test the difference between low- and high-risk group, stratified at

Table 10.2. Major metrics used to score machine learning models.

	Metric	Best score	Purpose
Regression	Maximum error	0	Captures the worst-case error
	Root mean square error (RMSE)	0	Emphasizes extreme values and outliers.
	Mean squared logarithmic error	0	Recommended for exponential targets, e.g., tumor size
	Mean absolute percentage error	0	Recommended when variables have different scales
	Median absolute error	0	Can deal with outliers
	Coefficient of determination (R^2)	1	Measures the scatter around the best fit
Classification	Accuracy	1	Measures correct predictions being positive or negative
	Precision	1	Measures the correct positive predictions
	Recall/sensitivity/true positive rate	1	Measures the ability to detect positive classes
	Specificity/true negative rate	1	Measures the ability to avoid false alarm
	Area under the curve (AUC)	1	Includes sensitivity and specificity, the most popular classification score
	F1-score	1	Includes precision and recall. Recommended to replace AUC when data is imbalanced [35]
Survival	Harrell's c-index	1	Most common survival models score
	Uno's c-index	1	Recommended when the amount of censoring is high [36]
	Log-rank statistics between risk groups		Easier to interpret

the median probability or pre-defined thresholds [39, 51]. Alternatively one can use the Brier score or time-dependent receiver-operating-characteristic curves [60].

Limitations of AUC. While AUC is the most popular metric for radiotherapy outcome studies, it should be kept in mind that it is a general measure of discriminatory ability of a classifier, and does not indicate clinical utility per se. There are clinical applications in which a predictive model with a relatively low AUC can be highly relevant, particularly if the classifier allows specific high- or low-risk groups to be carved out for which alternative treatment approaches are available. In that case accuracy in specific groups of particularly high (for treatment intensification) or low-risk (for de-escalation) is more applicable. Particularly for prediction of less frequent events AUC becomes less relevant, and the precision-recall curve is recommended as a more informative metric [61].

10.4 Practical considerations—building models for radiation oncology

Building a machine learning model is a multistep process made up of data pre-processing, feature selection, hyperparameter tuning, and parameter calibration. A major concern in this process is *overfitting*, which is common as models usually contain many more parameters than can be informatively constrained by the available data, enabling the model to simply learn the outcomes in the training data. Overfitting makes the model too sensitive to the training data such that its performance on unseen data decreases, meaning that it has high *variance*. In contrast, underfitted models lack fidelity and fail to capture signals inherent in the data (*bias*). Overfitting is not only relevant for model tuning but needs consideration in the entire model building process. To find the model with the highest performance (low bias, low variance) all aspects need to be considered, from data selection and preparation, sampling, model generation to scoring.

10.4.1 Input data

Features can be *categorical, ordinal,* or *continuous*. In ordinal variables the order of the categories is relevant such as in performance status or other disease-specific classifications. Ordinal features can be taken into account by assigning integers to each category based on the order, but it should be noted that in strictly linear models this can enforce a relationship between the different ordinal levels that might not be representative. Categorical features with more than two variables, such as race or tumor histology, need encoding to be processed by predictive models. *One-hot-encoding* is a common method in which each level of a categorical feature becomes a binary feature itself.

In radiotherapy outcome prediction features are roughly divided into *clinical* variables, i.e., patient and disease-specific factors, *image-based* predictors and *dosimetric* factors, which are defined by the radiation dose distribution and can theoretically be modified to change outcome. Care should be taken with assumptions that often pre-exist within the data, such as disease-specific composite scores (Child–Pugh Score or ALBI in liver disease for example) that are based on laboratory values, or nonlinear transformations of dose (see section 10.2).

In radiotherapy outcome modeling we are often building on datasets that have been previously published as clinical studies. In the ensuing statistical analysis continuous variables, particularly biomarkers, are often binned to increase robustness, for example as above/below median. While this might be indicated for smaller sample sizes [62], manual binning can lead to a significant loss in performance. Including the underlying continuous values enables algorithms to find an appropriate representation themselves. If data needs to be binned Hartemink's pairwise mutual information is superior to manual binning [63].

Imputation. Complete datasets, where all feature values are known for all patients, are scarce. Excluding patients with missing data reduces the sample size and can lead to bias. Missingness of data, i.e. if values are *missing-at-random* or not, has to be studied in the initial data exploration. *Informative missingness* in which the patterns of missing data are related to the outcome, can occur particularly in medical datasets and leads to bias. *Imputation* on the other hand replaces missing values with statistical estimates. Simple methods replace the missing value with a random selection from other samples or by the mean or median (for random forests) of all samples. Imputers available in most ML packages can use regression to predict missing values from the other features, which may prevent bias and noise of random selection. Note that data imputation should be done separately on the training and testing set to prevent data snooping. Data imputation can be useful in radiotherapy outcome prediction as often heavily correlated features exist such as tumor properties (stage, size, number of lesions).

If there is a large amount of data missing, Bayesian networks (BNs) should be considered. BNs are probabilistic graph models (nodes, edges) that encode a joint probability distribution among key factors and can be used to explore and present causal relationships between these key factors and final outcomes in an interpretable manner [33, 62, 64]. Due to their probabilistic nature they are very suited to modeling the noise that is inherent in clinical data, and they handle missing values very well through marginalization techniques.

10.4.2 Feature importance and selection

Models with a large number of features are prone to overfitting and loss of generalizability. Feature selection reduces the feature set by removing redundant and irrelevant features. A preliminary method is correlation analysis. This can be followed by identifying outcome-relevant features using feature importance, quantified as difference in model score with and without the feature. Alternatively, feature importance can be determined as change in the score after random shuffling of the feature values, named *permutation importance.* Permutation importance corrects for differences between continuous and categorical variables and is better suited when the model has mixed types of variables [65]. Permutation importance is often used in post-hoc analysis of complex models to understand model construction [57, 66].

Based on the feature importance, or feature permutation importance, the optimal feature set can be selected using iterative stepwise forward selection or backward elimination processes. The former starts with an empty feature set, measures the importance of every feature, and adds the most important feature to the feature set, iterating until all features are added. The latter conversely starts with a complete feature set and removes the least important features iteratively.

Simple and fast algorithms such as support vector machines and random forests are often used in a preliminary step to select relevant features [36]. In addition to the stepwise approaches, criterion-based methods use information theory to remove features with no or minimal information. Two major criteria for penalizing large models are the Akaike and the Bayesian Information Criteria [67, 68].

10.4.3 Tuning hyperparameters

Prior to fitting the model to the data, the model structure has to be defined, which is controlled by hyperparameters. In neural networks for instance, the edge weights are calibrated to fit the data but the hyperparameters such as the number of hidden layers and the number of nodes in each layer need to be defined first. Tuning hyperparameters is the process of finding the values that optimize the learning process and adjust the complexity of the model. It plays an important role in *regularization* and improves model generalization.

Each learning algorithm has its own hyperparameters, table 10.1 defines the major hyperparameters of common learning algorithms under 'Design considerations.' Usually, a simple grid search is used for tuning but better search methods such as random search and Bayesian optimization can be implemented to tune hyperparameters in case of large search spaces or demanding learning algorithms such as neural networks.

10.4.4 Resampling: cross-validation and bootstrapping

During model training, its parameters are calibrated to fit the data, relying on mathematical optimization to find the best score. Yet optimal scores do not imply predictive power. Models must be able to predict data outside the training set. Therefore, training a generalizable model needs two datasets, one for training and another for testing. The associated scores are referred to as train and test scores, or interchangeably internal and external scores.

Resampling techniques build subsets of samples *from the training data* to estimate model performance and robustness. Variables with high variance make the training scores sensitive to the data in the training set. Therefore multiple resampling is usually required to develop a robust model, yielding a distribution of results that can be aggregated and used to evaluate optimal choices and estimate uncertainty. The two main resampling methods are *cross-validation* and the *bootstrap*.

In k-fold cross-validation the data is partitioned into k groups: (k-1) groups are used for training and 1 group for testing. The process repeats k times. Although 10-fold cross-validation is common, the selection of k should consider the sample size and balance of data. In general, increasing the number of folds decreases the bias of the model, but increases the variance, i.e. making it more accurate but also more variable. For small sample sizes very small k values of 2 or 3 can also increase variance due to random sampling effects. Random splitting does not control for the frequency of the outcome in question—if the data is imbalanced *stratified splitting* should be used to include enough samples from each class in each of the k folds. However, this makes the assumption that later during evaluation the frequency of outcomes will be similar, and can lead to overly optimistic training scores if that is not the case. In leave-one-out cross-validation k equals the number of samples, though this procedure is computationally expensive for large datasets and has been shown to yield similar results to 10-fold cross-validation [69].

Bootstrapping is another resampling method where a new dataset is generated by drawing a random sample from the original dataset with replacement. In bootstrapping, the same sample could be selected multiple times and some other samples could be ignored but can still perform well if repeated enough times (typically hundreds to thousands depending on the original dataset). Minority oversampling can be used here to correct for class imbalance during the drawing process [36].

Variables with high variance make the internal training scores sensitive to the selection of samples in all resampling techniques. Multiple resampling is usually required to develop a robust model, where the average score becomes a measure of the predictive performance of the model. This can be achieved using *repeated* bootstrapping or cross-validation, which increases the precision of the parameter estimates while maintain small bias. For cross-validation this process is called *Monte-Carlo cross-validation* or *shuffle-split cross-validation* [35, 70, 71].

10.4.5 Nested cross-validation and final model selection

There is no one approach for combining feature selection, hyperparameter tuning and parameter calibration. Each step can be performed independently but this could yield suboptimal models. A more integrated approach can be achieved with *nested cross-validation* [62], see figure 10.1 for an overview of the process. As the name indicates, nested cross-validation has inner and outer loops. The outer loop splits the data into an internal set to develop the model and an external set to test it separately. In the inner loop, feature selection followed by hyperparameter tuning are performed using only the training dataset. At each iteration of hyperparameter tuning, the train dataset is partitioned again into internal training and internal testing sets to cross-validate the model at given hyperparameter values. The output

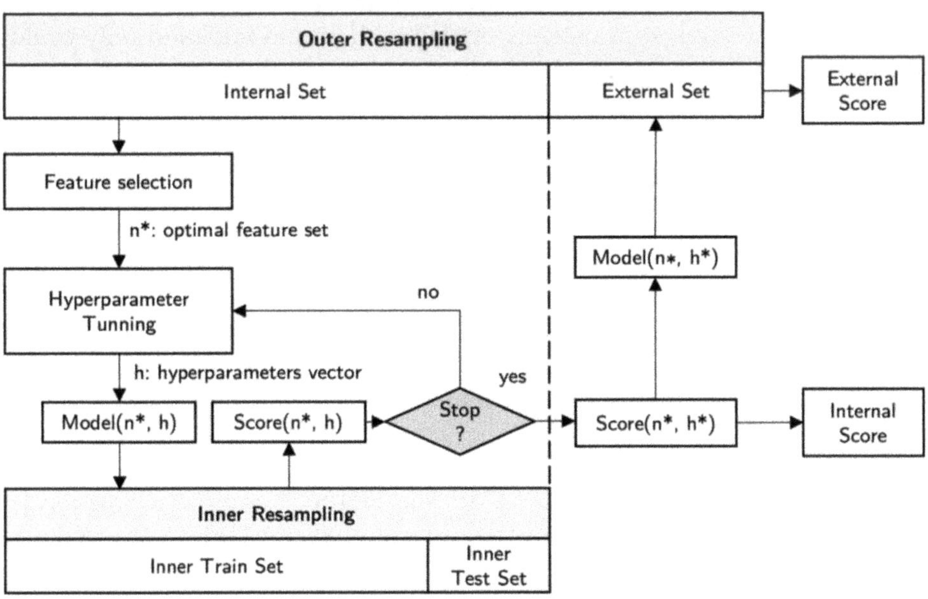

Figure 10.1. Workflow of the nested cross-validation framework used for model development.

of the inner loop is a model (choice of features and hyperparameters), which is then evaluated on the external dataset and its score recorded.

This repeated process, or a similarly repeated bootstrap, generates a large number of models, defined by a set of features and hyperparameters, equal to the number of iterations. Selecting a final model can be straightforward if one emerges as a dominant contender in the process, but can be difficult if the chosen models are very heterogeneous. It is advisable to not only use the average external score achieved, but also the variability of this score and the number of features to increase model robustness. Alternatively, one can set a fixed frequency threshold and include all models picked often enough in an ensemble model, which may enhance the model performance on new datasets particularly if the variance of available data is high. This has been shown to improve performance of different bootstrapped models chosen from DVH parameters [39].

10.4.6 Model validation

The reliability of predictive models increases with proper validation, however, the optimal procedure can depend on the size of the dataset and the purpose of the study. While often validation aims to estimate the ability of the model to generalize to unseen data, sometimes the actual purpose of the study is to evaluate the added predictive value of a given feature (i.e., additional imaging or a new biomarker) or to compare structurally different models to study which one performs best in capturing the information contained in the data.

The strongest validation is when the model is evaluated on a completely independent dataset. This could be a dataset from a different center or maybe even from a patient population with different characteristics. For example a model trained to predict survival in patients treated with chemo-radiation only could be evaluated by predicting pathologic complete response in those treated with chemo-radiation followed by surgery [51], providing a strong case for generalizable predictive power.

Less stringent is when one existing dataset is randomly split before model training [39]. The value of this hold-out techniques versus only performing internal validation is frequently discussed. When the number of samples is low it can be argued that every datapoint is needed for model building. Withholding data can lead to pessimistic bias as the model is not trained to its full capacity. Furthermore a test set represents a single evaluation of the model and cannot characterize the uncertainty in the results. Particularly if repeated internal training scores differ greatly from the validation score, it could be a situation where different test sets provide very different results. Sometimes dataset splitting and hold-out provides little additional information beyond the apparent performance evaluated through proper internal validation techniques [72]. The TRIPOD criteria (see section 10.6) provide more information on categorization of studies based on the underlying data.

10.5 Including dose distributions into data-driven outcome models

Compared to other predictors such as images and clinical features, dose distributions are very specific to radiotherapy, and a multitude of methods have been explored to include them into outcome models. While the classical NTCP models provide DVH-reduction formalisms and parameters weighing high- and low-dose regions (see section 10.2), data-driven models do not have such restrictions.

The most straightforward approach is to include all DVH points themselves as features. This leads to a large number of highly collinear predictors, not only *within* each organ but also among organs such as lung and heart, in which case parameter and model selection becomes paramount. A reasonable approach is to perform simple uni-variate correlation analyses of all DVH variables with the outcome in question, apply a Bonferroni correction, and use the DVH variable with the lowest p value per structure in further multi-variate modeling [39]. Otherwise penalized regression techniques, principal component analysis, genetic algorithms or more advanced deep learning approaches can also be used to manage feature collinearity [67, 73].

However such methods, particularly the selection of single DVH points per structure, can not only miss valuable information in the data, but also reduce the utility of the model in adapting treatment plans. Single DVH points might not comprehensively evaluate the effect of a treatment plan and optimization algorithms can sidestep them in ways that might not improve outcome.

Neural network structures have been used to include all DVH points, while leveraging the fact that they are highly correlated. Bi-directional long short-term memory structures have been shown to enable incorporating the entire DVH [30]. Bi-directionality is required as information decays along the recurrent network structure, and otherwise either the low- or high-dose region would be inherently weighed higher.

These methods still work with the dose-volume histogram as underlying data, which is a reduction of the full three-dimensional dose distribution. Feature extraction techniques from radiomics have been adapted to extract spatial dose metrics, sometimes referred to as *dosiomics* [71, 74, 75]. These features, such as dose-circumference histograms or 3D moment invariants can represent more information than included in DVHs.

The most advanced way to include the three-dimensional dose distribution is directly via convolutional neural networks. This requires registration of doses to a common reference anatomy to enable the network to learn locations of consistent dose patterns associated with a specific outcome. This technique has been implemented using multi-path neural networks that include clinical features to outcomes after SBRT for liver cancer [76, 77].

10.5.1 Voxel-based analysis

Voxel-based analysis (VBA) is a method to analyze three-dimensional dose distributions and identify local dose–response patterns [78, 79]. This methodology adequately accounts for non-dosimetric covariates and the multiple comparisons due to the large number of voxels. VBA can localize dose-sensitive regions correlated to a specific toxicity and the resulting patterns highlight the inhomogeneous radiation sensitivity of organs [80]. Various studies have utilized VBA for different organs and toxicities, including prostate, brain, lung and head-and-neck cancer [78, 81, 83].

The first and most important step of VBA is spatial normalization of dose distributions to a common coordinate system (CCS) [84], which can be either a digital phantom or a real patient image. In the next step a statistical analysis is performed that takes into account non-dosimetric covariates for the spatially normalized dose maps. For this purpose a generalized linear model is constructed for each voxel separately, using the dose as the dependent variable. The appropriate test statistic, e.g., a T statistic for comparison of two groups, is calculated and filtered. Next a permutation algorithm is applied that randomizes the variables at a patient level and calculates a separate T statistic map for each random permutation. The original T statistic can then be compared against the distribution of maximum T values of all the random permutations, which addresses the multiple comparison problem posed by the very large number of voxels.

10.6 Model reporting: TRIPOD and study analysis plans

Many prediction models have been developed but few of them are used in clinical practice [85], often due to poor standards in reporting model development and validation. In a three day meeting in 2011, methodologists, health care professionals, and journal editors collected and revised an extensive list of items needed for accurate reporting of predictive models and combined them into 22 essential items, forming the TRIPOD statement [86] (Transparent Reporting of a Multivariable Prediction Model for Individual Prognosis or Diagnosis). The complete checklist with detailed explanations can be found in [87] and has become a guideline for adequately reporting predictive models. A shortened list has been recommended for abstracts [88], which contains 12 items describing model development, external validation, the incremental value of adding predictors, and model updating.

The TRIPOD statement emphasizes model validation and provenance of data, classifying studies into four different types similarly to clinical trials, outlined in table 10.3. The publication of the TRIPOD statement had a positive impact on the practice of model development and validation in some respects, as the fraction of studies using external validation has increased and feature selection is described more completely [89]. Nevertheless, the overall reporting quality is still poor, especially regarding the proper description of the characteristics of the study population and the calibration between absolute predicted and observed outcomes.

The TRIPOD guidelines are currently under-used in radiotherapy outcome modeling, even though most aspects clearly apply. This is attributed to the fact that TRIPOD has been written and formulated from the perspective of regression-based predictive modeling approaches, so the terminology differs in some aspects and examples focus on regression. Therefore TRIPOD-ML has been recently launched to develop a statement specific to machine learning [90].

Table 10.3. Types of predictive model validation as classified by Collins *et al* [86].

Study Type	Description
Type 1 (a, b)	The model is developed using the entire dataset and is validated on the same set (type 1a) or another set obtained by resampling the data (type 1b).
Type 2 (a, b)	The data is split into two groups. One group is used for development and the other for validation based on either random (type 2a) or non-random splits (type 2b).
Type 3	Separate datasets, e.g., from different trials, used for development and validation.
Type 4	Validation of an existing, published model using a new dataset.

10.6.1 Study analysis plans

A significant concern for trust in models is when multiple models are developed in parallel or some calibration aspects or metrics are modified when validating with an external dataset. To increase transparency, it is strongly suggested that the scope and methods in a study analysis plan (SAP) are published before conducting data analysis and validation [91]. This measure, which is similar to the pre-registration of clinical trial protocols that define population and endpoints, prevents optimistic bias in model selection. SAPs can be easily published in public repositories such as the Open Science Foundation (OSF, https://osf.io/dashboard) to obtain a digital objective identifier and can be cited in the corresponding paper. The SAP should contain details on the study scope and analysis, such as variables and parameterization, handling of missing data, data resampling techniques, details on statistical analyses, and the validation procedure and metrics. For examples on SAPs for predictive models see references [92, 93].

10.7 Conclusion and future challenges

Precision radiation therapy needs truly personalized outcome models. The approaches and examples reviewed in this chapter show that there is enormous potential in these models for radiation oncology. To reach clinical utility, outcome modelers have to overcome two major challenges: lack of comprehensiveness and questions about clinical utility. For decision making we need models that provide a comprehensive picture of outcome, covering tumor control, toxicities, and other eventual outcomes of interest, while current models usually have a narrow focus. In the clinical context the trade-off between accuracy and interpretability [94] is often cited, however we believe that robust, well validated models with clinical utility will overcome such scrutiny. Predictive models built on information about dose distributions, be it DVH points or more advanced techniques (section 10.5), have not shown to be predictive for radiotherapy treatment planning as of now. It is unknown if optimizing patient dose distributions based on these models would actually improve outcome.

For radiotherapy specifically the integration of genetic information into outcome models has been lacking, which can characterize a large part of the heterogeneity among patients [36, 95, 98]. The integration of radiotherapy with novel biological agents will present another related challenge—the constant evolution of adjuvant therapies and shifting treatment paradigms will lead to models and their underlying data becoming outdated ever more rapidly. This will require more data sharing among centers, faster model updates and prospective validation to maintain clinical applicability.

References

[1] Okunieff P, Morgan D, Niemierko A and Suit H D 1995 Radiation dose–response of human tumors *Radiat. Oncol. Biol.* **32** 1227–37

[2] Ohri N *et al* 2012 Modeling local control after hypofractionated stereotactic body radiation therapy for stage I non-small cell lung cancer: a report from the elekta collaborative lung research group *Int. J. Radiat. Oncol. Biol. Phys.* **84** e379–84

[3] Ohri N *et al* 2021 Local control after stereotactic body radiation therapy for liver tumors *Int. J. Radiat. Oncol. Biol. Phys.* **110** 188–95

[4] McMahon S J 2019 The linear quadratic model: usage, interpretation and challenges *Phys. Med. Biol.* **64** 01TR01-25

[5] Dale R G 1985 The application of the linear-quadratic dose-effect equation to fractionated and protracted radiotherapy *Br. J. Radiol.* **58** 515–28

[6] Fowler J F 2010 21 years of biologically effective dose *Br. J. Radiol.* **83** 554–68

[7] Fowler J F and Dale R G 2010 When is a 'BED' not a 'BED'?-When it is an EQD2: in regard to Buyyounouski *et al* (*Int. J. Radiat. Oncol. Biol. Phys.* 2010;76:1297–1304) *Int. J. Radiat. Oncol. Biol. Phys.* **78** 640–41

[8] Thames H D, Peters L T, Withers H R and Fletcher G H 1983 Accelerated fractionation vs hyperfractionation: rationales for several treatments per day *Int. J. Radiat. Oncol. Biol. Phys.* **9** 127–38

[9] Joiner M C and van der Kogel A 2016 *Basic Clinical Radiobiology.* (London: Hodder Arnold)

[10] van Leeuwen C M *et al* 2018 The alfa and beta of tumours: a review of parameters of the linear-quadratic model, derived from clinical radiotherapy studies *Radiat. Oncol.* **13** 96–11

[11] Kirkpatrick J P, Meyer J J and Marks L B 2008 The linear-quadratic model is inappropriate to model high dose per fraction effects in radiosurgery *Semin. Radiat. Oncol.* **18** 240–43

[12] Astrahan M 2008 Some implications of linear-quadratic-linear radiation dose–response with regard to hypofractionation *Med. Phys.* **35** 4161–72

[13] Tomé W A 2009 Universal survival curve and single fraction equivalent dose: useful tools in understanding potency of ablative radiotherapy: in regard to Parks *et al* (*Int. J. Radiat. Oncol. Biol. Phys.* 2008;**72**:1620–1621) *Int. J. Radiat. Oncol. Biol. Phys.* **73** 1286

[14] Guckenberger M *et al* 2013 Applicability of the linear-quadratic formalism for modeling local tumor control probability in high dose per fraction stereotactic body radiotherapy for early stage non-small cell lung cancer *Radiother. Oncol. J. Eur. Soc. Ther. Radiol. Oncol.* **109** 13–20

[15] Shuryak I, Carlson D J, Brown J M and Brenner D J 2015 High-dose and fractionation effects in stereotactic radiation therapy: analysis of tumor control data from 2965 patients *Radiother. Oncol.* **115** 327–34

[16] Tree A C, Khoo V S, van As N J and Partridge M 2014 Is biochemical relapse-free survival after profoundly hypofractionated radiotherapy consistent with current radiobiological models? *Clin. Oncol.* **26** 216–29

[17] Klement R J *et al* 2020 Estimation of the α/β ratio of non-small cell lung cancer treated with stereotactic body radiotherapy *Radiother. Oncol.* **142** 210–16

[18] Vargo J A *et al* 2021 Head and neck Tumor control probability: radiation dose–volume effects in stereotactic body radiation therapy for locally recurrent previously-irradiated head and neck cancer: report of the AAPM working group *Int. J. Radiat. Oncol. Biol. Phys.* **110** 137–46

[19] Sahgal A *et al* 2021 Spinal cord dose tolerance to stereotactic body radiation therapy *Int. J. Radiat. Oncol. Biol. Phys.* **110** 124–36

[20] Munro T R 2008 The relation between tumour lethal doses and the radiosensitivity of tumour cells *Br. J. Radiol.* **34** 246–51

[21] Willers H and Held K D 2006 Introduction to clinical radiation biology *Hematol. Oncol. Clin. North Am.* **20** 1–24

[22] Bentzen S M 1992 Steepness of the clinical dose-control curve and variation in the *in vitro* radiosensitivity of head and neck squamous cell carcinoma *Int. J. Radiat. Biol.* **61** 417–23

[23] Dawson L A, Eccles C and Craig T 2009 Individualized image guided iso-NTCP based liver cancer SBRT *Acta Oncol.* **45** 856–64

[24] Cozzi L, Buffa F M and Fogliata A 2009 Comparative analysis of dose volume histogram reduction algorithms for normal tissue complication probability calculations *Acta Oncol.* **39** 165–71

[25] Marks L B, Ten Haken R K and Martel M K 2010 Guest editors introduction to QUANTEC: a users guide *Radiat. Oncol. Biol.* **76** S1–2

[26] Marks L B *et al* 2010 Use of normal tissue complication probability models in the clinic *Int. J. Radiat. Oncol. Biol. Phys.* **76** S10–9

[27] Grimm J *et al* 2021 High dose per fraction, hypofractionated treatment effects in the clinic (HyTEC): an overview *Int. J. Radiat. Oncol. Biol. Phys.* **110** 1–10

[28] Constine L S *et al* 2019 Pediatric normal tissue effects in the clinic (PENTEC): an int. collaboration to analyse normal tissue radiation dose-volume response relationships for paediatric cancer patients *Clin. Oncol.* **31** 199–207

[29] Moiseenko V *et al* 2020 A primer on dose–response data modeling in radiation therapy *Int. J. Radiat. Oncol. Biol. Phys.* **110** 11–20

[30] Zhu C *et al* 2020 A novel deep learning model using dosimetric and clinical information for grade 4 radiotherapy-induced lymphopenia prediction *Phys. Med. Biol.* **65** 035014

[31] Yu H *et al* 2019 Machine learning to build and validate a model for radiation pneumonitis prediction in patients with non-small cell lung cancer *Clin. Cancer Res.* **25** 4343–50

[32] Everson R M and Fieldsend J E 2006 Multi-class ROC analysis from a multi-objective optimisation perspective *Pattern Recogn. Lett.* **27** 918–27

[33] Luo Y *et al* 2018 A multiobjective Bayesian networks approach for joint prediction of tumor local control and radiation pneumonitis in nonsmall-cell lung cancer (NSCLC) for response-adapted radiotherapy *Med. Phys.* **45** 3980–95

[34] Hosmer D W, Lemeshow S and Sturdivant R X 2016 (Wiley Series in Probability and Statistics) (New York: Wiley) pp 269–311

[35] Deist T M *et al* 2018 Machine learning algorithms for outcome prediction in (chemo) radiotherapy: an empirical comparison of classifiers *Med. Phys.* **45** 3449–59

[36] Cui S, Luo Y, Tseng H, Haken R K T and Naqa I E 2019 Combining handcrafted features with latent variables in machine learning for prediction of radiation-induced lung damage *Med. Phys.* **46** 2497–511
[37] Kim S, Kim K, Choe J, Lee I and Kang J 2020 Improved survival analysis by learning shared genomic information from pan-cancer data *Bioinformatics* **36** i389–398
[38] Rokach L 2010 Ensemble-based classifiers *Artif. Intell. Rev.* **33** 1–39
[39] Thor M *et al* 2020 Modeling the impact of cardio-pulmonary irradiation on overall survival in NRG Oncology trial RTOG 0617 *Clin Cancer Res.* **2627** 2019
[40] Coates J T T, Pirovano G and Naqa I E 2021 Radiomic and radiogenomic modeling for radiotherapy: strategies, pitfalls, and challenges *J. Med. Imaging* **8** 031902
[41] Sahiner B *et al* 2019 Deep learning in medical imaging and radiation therapy *Med. Phys.* **46** e1–36
[42] Han W *et al* 2019 Deep transfer learning and radiomics feature prediction of survival of patients with high-grade gliomas *Am. J. Neuroradiol.* **41** 40–8
[43] Yu J *et al* 2020 Lymph node metastasis prediction of papillary thyroid carcinoma based on transfer learning radiomics *Nat. Commun.* **11** 4807
[44] Hettal L *et al* 2020 Radiomics method for the differential diagnosis of radionecrosis versus progression after fractionated stereotactic body radiotherapy for brain oligometastasis *Radiat. Res.* **193** 471–80
[45] Park Y W *et al* 2021 Differentiation of recurrent glioblastoma from radiation necrosis using diffusion radiomics with machine learning model development and external validation *Sci. Rep.* **11** 2913
[46] Cai J *et al* 2020 A radiomics model for predicting the response to bevacizumab in brain necrosis after radiotherapy *Clin. Cancer Res.* **26** 5438–47
[47] Mattonen S A *et al* 2016 Detection of local cancer recurrence after stereotactic ablative radiation therapy for lung cancer: physician performance versus radiomic assessment *Int. J. Radiat. Oncol. Biol. Phys.* **94** 1121–128
[48] Cha K H *et al* 2017 Bladder cancer treatment response assessment in CT using radiomics with deep-learning *Sci Rep.* **7** 8738
[49] Chen X *et al* 2017 Assessment of treatment response during chemoradiation therapy for pancreatic cancer based on quantitative radiomic analysis of daily CTs: an exploratory study *PLoS One* **12** e0178961
[50] Hosny A *et al* 2018 Deep learning for lung cancer prognostication: a retrospective multi-cohort radiomics study *PLoS Med.* **15** e1002711
[51] Xu Y *et al* 2019 Deep learning predicts lung cancer treatment response from serial medical imaging *Clin. Cancer Res.* **25** 3266–75
[52] Dercle L *et al* 2020 Reinventing radiation therapy with machine learning and imaging bio-markers (radiomics): state-of-the-art, challenges and perspectives *Methods* **188** 44–60
[53] Boldrini L, Bibault J-E, Masciocchi C, Shen Y and Bittner M-I 2019 Deep learning: a review for the radiation oncologist *Front. Oncol.* **9** 977
[54] Gourgou-Bourgade S *et al* 2015 Guidelines for time-to-event end point definitions in breast cancer trials: results of the DATECAN initiative (definition for the assessment of time-to-event endpoints in CANcer trials) *Ann. Oncol.* **26** 2505–506
[55] Wu X *et al* 2017 Personalized prognostic prediction models for breast cancer recurrence and survival incorporating multidimensional data *JNCI J. Natl Cancer Inst.* **109** djw314

[56] Ishwaran H, Kogalur U B, Chen X and Minn A J 2011 Random survival forests for high-dimensional data *Stat. Anal. Data. Min.* **4** 115–32
[57] Peeken J C *et al* 2019 Combining multimodal imaging and treatment features improves machine learning-based prognostic assessment in patients with glioblastoma multiforme *Cancer Med-US* **8** 128–36
[58] Demler O V, Pencina M J and D'Agostino R B 2012 Misuse of delong test to compare AUCs for nested models *Stat. Med.* **31** 2577–87
[59] Pepe M S, Kerr K F, Longton G and Wang Z 2013 Testing for improvement in prediction model performance *Stat. Med.* **32** 1467–82
[60] Chen H-C, Kodell R L, Cheng K F and Chen J J 2012 Assessment of performance of survival prediction models for cancer prognosis *BMC Med. Res. Methodol.* **12** 102
[61] Ozenne B, Subtil F and Maucort-Boulch D 2015 The precision–recall curve overcame the optimism of the receiver operating characteristic curve in rare diseases *J. Clin. Epidemiol.* **68** 855–9
[62] Luo Y *et al* 2019 Development of a fully cross-validated Bayesian network approach for local control prediction in lung cancer *IEEE Trans. Radiat. Plasma Med. Sci.* **3** 232–41
[63] Hartemink A J 2001 Principled computational methods for the validation discovery of genetic regulatory networks *Thesis* Massachusetts Institute of Technology
[64] Oh J H *et al* 2011 A Bayesian network approach for modeling local failure in lung cancer *Phys. Med. Biol.* **56** 1635–51
[65] Altmann A, Toloşi L, Sander O and Lengauer T 2010 Permutation importance: a corrected feature importance measure *Bioinformatics* **26** 1340–7
[66] Shew M, New J and Bur A M 2018 Machine learning to predict delays in adjuvant radiation following surgery for head and neck cancer *Otolaryngol. Head Neck Surg.* **160** 1058–64
[67] Mizutani T *et al* 2019 Optimization of treatment strategy by using a machine learning model to predict survival time of patients with malignant glioma after radiotherapy *J. Radiat. Res.* **60** 818–24
[68] Neath A A and Cavanaugh J E 2012 The Bayesian information criterion: background, derivation, and applications *Wiley Interdiscip. Rev. Comput. Stat.* **4** 199–203
[69] Molinaro A M, Simon R and Pfeiffer R M 2005 Prediction error estimation: a comparison of resampling methods *Bioinformatics* **21** 3301–7
[70] Dean J *et al* 2018 Incorporating spatial dose metrics in machine learning-based normal tissue complication probability (NTCP) models of severe acute dysphagia resulting from head and neck radiotherapy *Clin. Transl. Radiat. Oncol.* **8** 27–39
[71] Dean J A *et al* 2016 Normal tissue complication probability (NTCP) modelling using spatial dose metrics and machine learning methods for severe acute oral mucositis resulting from head and neck radiotherapy *Radiother. Oncol.* **120** 21–7
[72] Moons K G M *et al* 2014 Critical appraisal and data extraction for systematic reviews of prediction modelling studies: the CHARMS checklist *PLoS Med.* **11** e1001744
[73] Pan X *et al* 2020 Dosimetric predictors of patient-reported toxicity after prostate stereotactic body radiotherapy: analysis of full range of the dose–volume histogram using ensemble machine learning *Radiother. Oncol.* **148** 181–8
[74] Dean J A *et al* 2017 Normal tissue complication probability (NTCP) modelling of severe acute mucositis using a novel Oral mucosal surface organ at risk *Clin. Oncol.* **29** 263–73

[75] Gabryś H S, Buettner F, Sterzing F, Hauswald H and Bangert M 2018 Design and selection of machine learning methods using radiomics and dosiomics for normal tissue complication probability modeling of xerostomia *Front. Oncol.* **8** 35

[76] Ibragimov B *et al* 2019 Neural networks for deep radiotherapy dose analysis and prediction of liver SBRT outcomes *J. Biomed. Health Inform.* **23** 1821–33

[77] Ibragimov B *et al* 2018 Development of deep neural network for individualized hepatobiliary toxicity prediction after liver SBRT *Med. Phys.* **45** 4763–74

[78] Acosta O *et al* 2013 Voxel-based population analysis for correlating local dose and rectal toxicity in prostate cancer radiotherapy *Phys. Med. Biol.* **58** 2581–95

[79] Palma G, Monti S and Cella L 2020 Voxel-based analysis in radiation oncology: a methodological cookbook *Phys. Medica* **69** 192–204

[80] Palma G *et al* 2019 Spatial signature of dose patterns associated with acute radiation-induced lung damage in lung cancer patients treated with stereotactic body radiation therapy *Phys. Med. Biol.* **64** 155006

[81] Palma G *et al* 2019 Spatial dose patterns associated with radiation pneumonitis in a randomized trial comparing intensity-modulated photon therapy with passive scattering proton therapy for locally advanced non-small cell lung cancer *Int. J. Radiat. Oncol. Biol. Phys.* **104** 1124–32

[82] Monti S *et al* 2017 Voxel-based analysis unveils regional dose differences associated with radiation-induced morbidity in head and neck cancer patients *Sci. Rep.* **7** 7220

[83] Monti S *et al* 2020 A novel framework for spatial normalization of dose distributions in voxel-based analyses of brain irradiation outcomes *Phys. Medica* **69** 164–9

[84] Monti S, Pacelli R, Cella L and Palma G 2018 Inter-patient image registration algorithms to disentangle regional dose bioeffects *Sci Rep.* **8** 4915

[85] Steyerberg E W *et al* 2013 Prognosis research strategy (PROGRESS) 3: prognostic model research *PLoS Med.* **10** e1001381

[86] Collins G S, Reitsma J B, Altman D G and Moons K G 2015 Transparent reporting of a multivariable prediction model for individual prognosis or diagnosis (TRIPOD): the TRIPOD Statement *BMC Med.* **13** 1–10

[87] Moons K G M *et al* 2015 Transparent reporting of a multivariable prediction model for individual prognosis Or diagnosis (TRIPOD): explanation and elaboration *Ann. Intern. Med.* **162** W1

[88] Heus P *et al* 2020 Transparent reporting of multivariable prediction models in journal and conference abstracts: TRIPOD for abstracts *Ann. Intern. Med.* **173** 42–7

[89] Najafabadi A H Z *et al* 2020 TRIPOD statement: a preliminary pre-post analysis of reporting and methods of prediction models *Bmj Open* **10** e041537

[90] Collins G S and Moons K G M 2019 Reporting of artificial intelligence prediction models *Lancet* **393** 1577–9

[91] Thor M, Oh J H, Apte A P and Deasy J O 2020 Registering study analysis plans (SAPs) before dissecting your data—updating and standardizing outcome modeling *Frontiers Oncol* **10** 978

[92] Chamseddine I, Kim Y, Paganetti H and Grassberger C 2020 Predicting radiotherapy outcomes in hepatocellular carcinoma. https://osf.io/6pwgk

[93] Thor M and Deasy J 2018 The role of heart-related dose–volume metrics on overall survival in the RTOG 0617 clinical trial https://osf.io/hzsva

[94] Luo Y *et al* 2019 Balancing accuracy and interpretability of machine learning approaches for radiation treatment outcomes modeling *BJR|Open* **1** 20190021–12
[95] Lee S *et al* 2018 Machine learning on a genome-wide association study to predict late genitourinary toxicity after prostate radiation therapy *Int. J. Radiat. Oncol. Biol. Phys.* **101** 128–35
[96] Naqa I E *et al* 2018 Modeling of locoregional control in hepatocellular carcinoma after stereotactic body radiation therapy by integrating clinical and immune cell profiles *Int. J. Radiat. Oncol. Biol. Phys.* **102** S7
[97] Scott J G *et al* 2020 Personalizing radiotherapy prescription dose using genomic markers of radiosensitivity and normal tissue toxicity in non-small cell lung cancer *J. Thorac. Oncol.* **16** 428–38
[98] Cui S, Haken R K T and Naqa I E 2021 Integrating multi-omics information in deep learning architectures for joint actuarial outcome prediction in non-small-cell lung cancer patients after radiation therapy *Int. J. Radiat. Oncol. Biol. Phys.* **110** 893–904

Chapter 11

Challenges in artificial intelligence development of radiotherapy

Huanmei Wu and Jay S Patel

11.1 Radiomics: past, current, and future

Radiomics was first introduced in radiology, referring to the high-throughput extraction and analysis of high-dimensional radiographic images, in 2012 [1]. Examining radiographs and medical images using a simple eyeballing method was the most prominent method of interpreting the findings. However, radiomics driven by medical image analysis has grown exponentially, with an increased number of pattern recognition tools and an increase in dataset sizes. The initial focus of radiomics is to improve image analysis using a large amount (200+) of extracted quantitative features of medical images, including computed tomography (CT), positron emission tomography (PET), and magnetic resonance imaging (MRI). The underlying hypothesis of radiomics will connect radiological images with proteomics and genomics [1–3]. Radiomics will not only identify the region of interest (ROI) for physicians but also integrate quantifiable content-based imaging information for advanced data mining and big data analysis [3].

Radiomics has many potential clinical applications [4, 5]. One of the earliest applications is to use radiomics from CT images to predict tumor shrinkage in non-small cell lung cancer (NSCLC) patients [6]. Texture analysis of the gray-scale image intensity in FDG-PET/CT and other imaging modalities provide additional predictive features, prognostic information, tumor heterogeneity, and the underlying biological mechanisms [7]. A subset of textual, shape- and intensity-based radiomic features from CT images can predict lung cancer patient survival, intratumoural heterogeneity, and risk of distant metastasis [8, 9]. Some features and prediction power can be cancer-type dependent [10]. Texture features extracted from joint FDG-PET/T1, FDG-PET/T2FS, and MRI scans were used in the early evaluation of lung metastasis risk in soft-tissue sarcomas (STSs) [11]. Other studies also applied radiomic texture analysis (TA) features of functional magnetic resonance imaging

doi:10.1088/978-0-7503-3339-9ch11

(fMRI) scans associated with tumor heterogeneity in predicting the regions of interest with the true functional activity or correlating with meaningful brain activity [12, 13].

Radiomics is a rapidly evolving field of research. There are four modern directions of radiomics in radiation oncology and radiology.

11.1.1 Multiparametric radiomics

The widely used image-based radiomics are textual features and regions of interest extracted from single images. Single image radiomics cannot capture the true underlying tissue characteristics with limited information available within the data, constraining the application of radiomics in various clinical settings. The multiparametric imaging radiomic framework (MPRAD) emerged which can extract the first- and second-order radiomic features from high-dimensional multi-parametric radiological datasets [14]. For example, multiparametric MRI includes diffusion imaging, MRI spectrography, PET scans, tomosynthesis (3D mammography), and various ultrasound procedures [15]. Multiparametric radiomics can be used for multiple diseases, such as breast cancer and strokes [14].

11.1.2 Multi-radiomics

As imaging features, i.e., are the phenotypes of the underlying biological mechanisms and gene sets for cell cycle phase, DNA recombination, or regulation of immune system process [1]. Imaging genomics or radiogenomics is another rising field of study associating imaging features with genomic data, thus, bridging imaging and genomics [16, 17]. As demonstrated in figure 11.1, in a study for the benefit of prediction of adjuvant chemotherapy, the researchers have not only used radiomic texture features derived from chest CT scans but also performed radiogenomic analysis over mRAN sequence data (i.e., the genomic data) for the underlying biological characteristics and radiopathomic analysis on the tissue images of corresponding surgical specimens [18].

Radiomics and radiogenomics correlate quantitative imaging features to genomic data, which are attractive research topics in prostate cancer [19]. For instance, studies showed that somatic mutations of tumors drive biological processes reflected in tumor phenotype, especially, in medical images [20, 21]. This connection between imaging phenotype and cancer genetics promoted the use of imaging-based biomarkers in the clinic. The traditional radiomics has been extended to the cutting edge multi-radiomics with heterogeneous biomedical information, combining imaging textual information, tumor complexity (staging, shape, size, etc), patient demographics, histology, genomics, proteomics, SNP, and single-cell data. For instance, Jiang *et al* applied machine learning (ML) models on combined dosimetric factors and radiomics features [22]. The study focused on five ROIs from the treatment planning CT images and five dosimetric factors from the dose-volume histograms. The image preprocessing and radiomics feature extraction calculated four categories of commonly used radiomics features, including shape features,

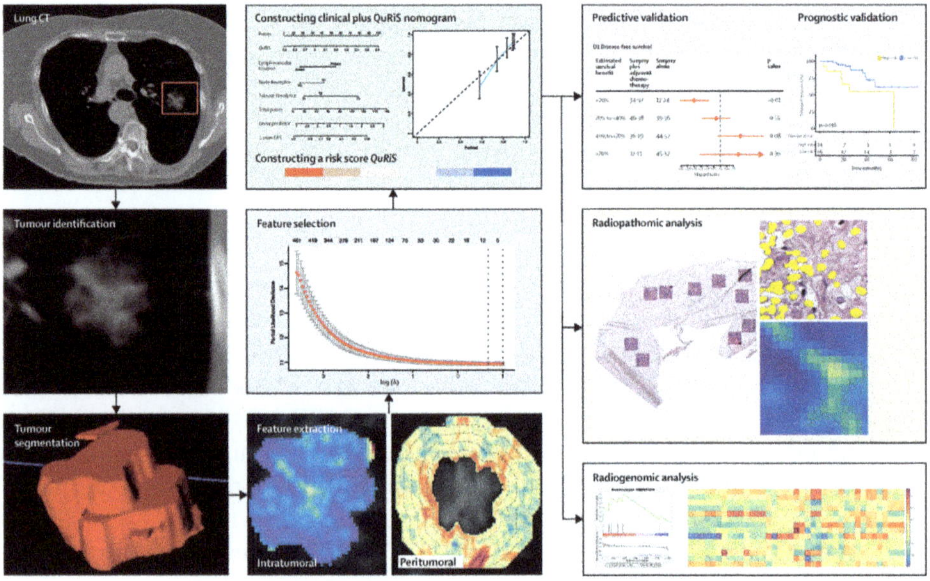

Figure 11.1. Sample project with association between radiomic, pathomic, and genomic data (from Vaidya *et al* 2020). Reprinted from The Lancet [18], copyright (2020), with permission from Elsevier.

intensity features, texture features, and Laplacian of Gaussian (LoG) filtered features, resulting in a total of 1924 features across all five ROIs.

11.1.3 Artificial intelligence (AI)-empowered radiomics

The complex big data from the modern multi-radiomics also promotes the cutting edge application of engineered algorithms, automatic deep-learning methods, and artificial intelligence methods to quantify both genotypic and phenotypic characters in tumors [20, 23, 24]. For example, the multiparametric deep-learning tissue signature model (MPDL) has applied multiparametric MRI to capture the brain texture, which could be potential biomarkers for distinguishing grade IV from grade II tumors as well as determining true-progression from pseudo-progression [23]. The study of Yu *et al* used machine learning methods to develop a generalized linear mixed model to predict radiation pneumonitis adverse events in NSCLC patients receiving thoracic radiotherapy [25]. The study integrated the expression levels of 30 inflammatory cytokines, patient demographic characteristics (e.g., gender or age), behavior attributes (e.g., smoking status), physiological functions (e.g., Karnofsky performance status scales), medical conditions (e.g., CVD or COPD), radiomics features (e.g., tumor volume and shape), dosimetric factors (e.g., lung or heart radiation doses), tumor information (e.g., clinical stages), and treatment approaches (e.g., chemotherapy). Machine learning helped to select the predictive GLM model that identified the combined cytokines and clinical variables for radiation pneumonitis prediction.

11.1.4 Precision radiotherapy

Emerging evidence has shown that precision radiotherapy for cancer patients is possible with recent advances in new radiotherapy technologies, panomics, radiomics and dosiomics [26]. For example, radiotherapy dose influenced the systemic activity of indoleamine 2,3-dioxygenase (IDO) in NSCLC. IDO has a significant impact on metastatic risk and overall survival, which can be a biomarker to optimize radiation dose in patients to improve outcomes [26]. In another study, secondary analysis of multi-radiomics using a weighted-support vector machine (SVM) classifier discovered circulating cytokine biomarkers to predict radiation-induced lung fibrosis (RILF) in NSCLC patients, along with other clinical parameters [27]. For head and neck cancer patients, pioneers have explored new ideas to have personalized treatment with an improved understanding of the phenotypic and genotypic differences between patients and their tumors. Genomics, radiomics, and mathematical modeling promise treatment personalization for patients with head and neck cancer, with improved radiotherapy outcomes while reducing complications [28].

11.2 AI and multi-radiomics as a hybrid way for AI development

The concept of the application of artificial intelligence (AI) to radiotherapy is not new in medicine. The initial applications were developed back in 1963 and 1973, where researchers attempted to create computer applications for the diagnosis of cancer [29, 30]. This enthusiasm reduced over time until recent years. With the new wave of machine learning (ML) and deep learning (DL), many researchers have been utilizing electronic health records, medical images, radiomics, multi-omics, and other heterogeneous biomedical information using advanced AI approaches for early prevention, screening, diagnosis, disease identification, biological characterization, treatment improvement, and toxicity reduction. The AI applications have spanned radiotherapy for brain, skin, lung, breast, and gastrointestinal cancers [31–35]. These applications are still in the process and validation phases. Despite the significant increase in the utilization of image process methods, the transition of the findings to the bedside is limited for the reasons given below.

First, most research has used single institution datasets that limit the generalizability of the study findings. Many factors, such as cultural, behavioral, and social determinants of health, can impact the collected data based on the patients' geographical regions. Thus, the validation datasets need to be from different institutions or clinics to improve the generalizability of the study findings. Next, the AI algorithms need to be retrained on the validation datasets if the AI performance are suboptimal. However, due to the strict HIPAA regulations, it is difficult to obtain large-scale datasets for AI applications from various regions.

Fortunately, the National Institutes of Health (NIH) have realized the challenges and led research data-sharing for secondary research. NIH requires funded investigators to publish their collection of imaging and clinical data. In addition, the

National Cancer Institute (NCI) has created the National Biomedical Image Archive software package to host cancer-related imaging data, the open-source, open-access The Cancer Imaging Archive (TCIA). It has helped research, development, and educational initiatives utilizing advanced medical imaging of cancer [36, 37]. There is a need for more initiatives in addition to TCIA for researchers to develop more advanced and high-performing AI algorithms [38].

Another bottleneck is obtaining manually labeled gold standard datasets as it is time-consuming and expensive, which requires clinical domain expertise. Next, there is a need to incorporate medical images, lab values, doctors' notes, nurse evaluations, and other relevant features. For example, clinical decision support systems diagnosis and treatment planning require besides images, radiographs, radiomics, and other clinically relevant features for optimized system performance. Last, the biopsy is still considered to be the gold standard for the diagnosis of chronic conditions, including cancer. AI algorithms helping clinicians with cancer diagnoses would be a liability issue for the clinicians without taking into consideration biopsy samples. A recent systemic review [39] on AI applications in radiomics concluded that the results of the current research studies on medical image processing are promising. However, they are still not mature enough to be implemented in the clinical setting. More validation studies are required that produce good generalizability with high accuracy to improve the diagnosis, treatment planning, and disease screening.

11.3 Ethics and regulations for artificial intelligence using biomedical informatics

As AI has attracted renewed attention in the last few years, many revolutionary changes have occurred from various industries with the applications of AI to our everyday lives. Google, Microsoft, Facebook, Twitter, Amazon, Apple, and other big companies have achieved tremendous success when it comes to automation, voice recognition, and personalized recommendations and care. For example, Amazon recommends personalized products based on your previous purchases or browsing histories [40]. Many translating services have been implemented in your smartphones or smart speakers at home. They can recognize your voice and convert it into text, which has been used in our daily life and advanced education [41, 42]. Google search will display the best search results based on the keywords. Tesla vehicles, equipped with advanced AI for vision and planning, make Autopilot self-driving systems possible [43, 44]. These are great examples of the successful applications of AI that frequently surround us.

Similarly, the use of AI in healthcare has also gained significant attention in the last few years. AI has pushed the boundaries of human performance and showed promising results that even experts cannot perform. For example, Google Health has developed prediction models to predict the onset of acute kidney injury before the injury occurs with high accuracy. Compared to the current medical practice, mostly kidney injury is only noticed after it has already occurred, such prediction models are of great use to prevent injuries. Next, it is now well known that after the implementation of electronic health records (EHR) to document patient information, there is a significant increase in the burnout rate among physicians and nurses. Since the last decade, many researchers have been working on converting EHR free-text data into a structured format and auto-fill features within the EHR to reduce the burden of the documentation process among physicians and nurses [45, 46]. Moreover, some studies have also demonstrated that AI could be used to predict the staffing needs and predict the revenue of the organizations to improve resource sharing [47]. An AI platform that enables doctors and oncologists to help ease conversations with terminally ill patients has also been developed [48].

However, the robustness of AI algorithms is not as effective in healthcare compared to the AI algorithms used in the above-described industries. Moreover, the deployment of AI tools for patient care is still in its infancy in healthcare. There are many reasons for healthcare to lag in optimal AI utilization and they are briefly described below.

Trust issues among experts: One of the major concerns of using AI for patient care is trust issues among clinicians, experts, and caregivers. Healthcare professionals are afraid that the AI systems will generate incorrect results, diagnoses, and treatment recommendations that will lead to injury or harm to their patients. For example, the failure of AI to notice tumors in radiographs or miss identifying cancer patients would lead to a delayed or missed diagnosis even though many human errors, without the involvement of AI, have caused injury. However, the way errors caused by humans versus AI would be viewed and reacted to differently [49–51].

Privacy concerns: It has been popular among interdisciplinary scientists to mine 'big data' in healthcare to generate evidence-based care for the last decade. Massive healthcare data, including the TCIA imaging repository [38], i2b2 dataset, and many others. They use large sample sizes, develop prediction models and learning health systems, and develop personalized diagnostic and treatment recommendations. Since the patients' data have been used widely by the researchers, concerns have been raised by patients, care providers, and others about the extensive use of patient information, which might violate patient privacy. Lawsuits have been filed based on data-sharing between large health systems and AI developments [52]. On the other hand, AI could predict the disease status of a patient without using their private information. For example, AI can diagnose a patients' Parkinson's Disease status by examining how they are using a computer mouse. Even though the patients' personal information has not been used, the patient may be concerned about their privacy [53–55].

Poor generalizability and bias: As we know, *garbage in, garbage out (GIGO)*. It is extremely important to have quality data for AI systems as they learn from the data. If the data entered in the AI system is biased, the outcome would be subjective as well. There are many real-life examples of discriminating artificial intelligence where the AI algorithms demonstrate biases and prejudices [56].

Example of racial bias in health a algorithm [57]: Researchers discovered that one widely used algorithm in the US healthcare system for health decisions has racial bias. Although race is not a variable in the algorithm, the algorithm assumed health costs represented health needs. However, statistics showed that black patients have lower average health costs than their white counterparts with the same medical conditions. The biased assumption induced a false conclusion that black patients are healthier than equally sick qhite patients. The biased outcome would make black patients lose out on critical care. Fortunately, it was caught by researchers. The algorithm was reformatted without the underlying incorrect assumption, reducing 80% of the biases and eliminating racism in predicting who needs extra care.

Currently, most AI systems are built based on EHR data. However, EHR data has certain limitations and data quality issues. There are many missing data, inaccurate diagnostic codes, and duplicated information presented in different sections of the EHR. If the AI system learns from the 'garbage' data, the result would be biased or inaccurate as well (GIGO) [58].

Moreover, most AI systems are developed using academic datasets, limited by the constrained population for data collection. The findings generated from such datasets cannot be generalized and applied to other people and scenarios. Similarly, if a speech-recognition AI system is used to transcribe encounter notes, the AI algorithm may not perform well for all providers, especially when a provider is of a race or accent underrepresented in training data.

Ethical issues: Racial discrimination is one of the most concerning ethical issues with using AI for healthcare. An algorithm designed to predict outcomes from genetic findings will be biased if there have been few (or no) genetic studies in certain populations. Unfortunately, the majority of genomics data are from the white population. For example, the Framingham Heart Study data has led to biased predictions of overestimated or underestimated cardiovascular risks in non-white populations [59, 60]. The intent behind the developed AI algorithm should also be considered and determined whether it is ethical or not. Uber's tool Greyball is designed to predict which ride hailers could be undercover law enforcement officers. However, the tool would allow drivers to identify and bypass local regulations [61].

Similarly, in healthcare, it is a concern that clinical decision support systems (CDSS) may also be programmed in a way that it recommends certain drugs, procedures, tests, or devices to increase the revenue of the hospital without clinicians being aware of it. There is always tension between the goals of improving health and generating revenue and profits. This tension must be acknowledged and considered while training AI algorithms. Some clinicians are also threatened and afraid of AI taking over their tasks and eventually their job. For example, in radiology, AI has already taken on a wide variety of tasks such as automatic lesion detection, predicting risk, and providing differential diagnosis and treatment planning. Hence, it is important to consider such concerns while designing AI algorithms.

11.4 Heterogeneous biomedical data management

There is heterogeneous biomedical information for personalized healthcare and precision radiotherapy. Managing these data from different institutes with various systems will be challenging. There are nationwide movements in addressing different tasks of AI applications in biomedical and healthcare domains. For example, the

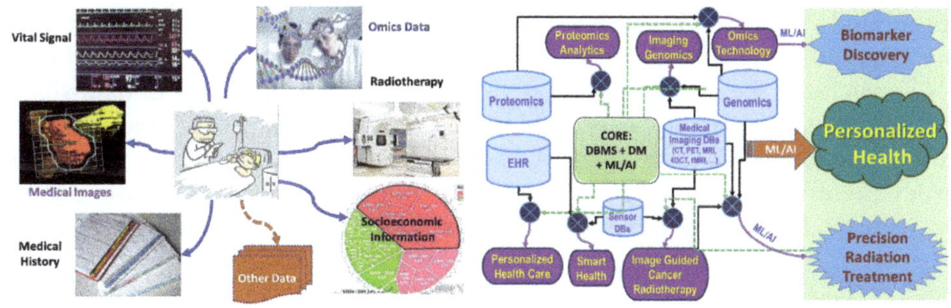

(a) A BMI bid data warehouse. (b) an Intelligent precision health framework.

Figure 11.2. Biomedical information (BMI) management and an intelligent precision health framework enabled by advanced ML/AI.

newly created Bridge to Artificial Intelligence (Bridge2AI) program by the NIH Common Fund will propel biomedical research forward and promote the adoption of AI applications for complex biomedical challenges beyond human intuition [62].

Figure 11.2(a) lists some specific biomedical information for patient care, which includes the medical records (most in EHRs), medical images (most stored in a secure file system), vital signals (most connected with electronic devices for real-time observations), omics data (which generated by high-throughput sequencing technology and stored separated by the principal investigators), treatment approaches (such as surgery, radiotherapy, chemotherapy, etc), patients' socioeconomic data (at personal, family or community levels, which is collected separately), and many other data. Each type of data includes hundreds of different variables. For example, medical images can be PET/SPECT, MRI, x-ray, CT, ultrasound, and other images. Each image type again can have sub-modalities. To give a specific example, the CT images used in radiotherapy can have diagnostic CT, planning CT, 4DCT, cone-beam CT (CBCT), and other CT. The CT can be 2D, 3D, and multidimensional. Each medical image quality is associated with a specific machine under various lighting and patient conditions. To make successful AI applications, these complicated biomedical data must be well integrated with common standards with well-structured descriptions.

Figure 11.2(b) gives examples of AI applications based on different available biomedical data, including biomarker discovery, personalized healthcare, and prediction radiotherapy. There is one fundamental challenge to integrating the data with the core database management systems (DBMS): common standards for different datasets from all institutes. Only after these data have been fully understood by the AI algorithm designers and developers, can the AI applications have the potential to be accurate, unbiased, and secured. There is a long way to go. There are still no standards available for most of the data types yet, including but not limited to omics data and social determinants of health.

Additional challenges come with health information exchange (HIE) across healthcare organizations, which allows healthcare professionals and patients to appropriately access and securely share a patient's medical information electronically. The Office of the National Coordinator for Health Information Technology (ONC) has listed the primary six types of HIE stakeholders for health data-sharing, including patient, primary care, specialist, laboratory, hospital, and pharmacy. During health information sharing, there are associated problems with patient privacy preservation, data quality checks, data ownership, sharing authorizations, data security during data transitions from one place to another and while staying at one organization, and many others.

11.5 Human harms due to AI

With the increased development of health-oriented AI tools and their implementation in healthcare, concerns exist that could lead to patient injury and medical liability. The existing laws in the US let the clinicians make the final diagnosis and treatment planning decisions. Therefore, AI may not be directly responsible for the AI malfunctioning or failures. However, there are still potential malpractice lawsuits that hospitals and clinicians can face while using AI technology for patient care. For example, physicians may be liable for not critically evaluating the outputs generated by the AI as, after all, clinicians are responsible for the diagnosis and treatment planning. AI tools are only responsible for making 'recommendations' to the clinicians and not the final diagnosis or treatment planning. Clinicians may also be liable for their decision to implement the AI system, and/or their employees' negligent treatment decisions using AI tools. Last, there could also be a product liability if the clinicians have been involved in developing and designing such systems.

There are thousands of lawsuits due to AI malfunctions in healthcare. These lawsuits were the results of both hardware and software AI system failures. For instance, the Da Vinci surgical system is designed to improve the precision in surgeries by using a minimally invasive approach. The Da Vinci system has been used to perform surgical removal of cancer tumors such as prostate, thyroid, and gastric cancer tumor removals [63, 64]. It has been reported that there have been 144 deaths, 1392 patient injuries, and 8061 device malfunctions reported which are the fault of the AI systems. It has also been reported that 14.7% reported cases had burnt or broken pieces of instruments fall into the patient, 8.6% involved unintended operation of the instruments, and 5% reported system errors [65].

It is an interesting and controversial topic of discussion because the ideal approach to compare the usefulness of such systems would be by comparing its performance with the manual work performed by the clinicians. For instance, comparing the errors made by the Da Vinci surgical system versus errors made by surgeons performing surgeries without the help of the Da Vinci surgical system. If the error rates are significantly lower when the AI systems are used compared to manual surgery work, then it is still better to use these systems despite the existing errors. One has to keep in mind that no system or human judgment is perfect, and just because the 'system' malfunctioned, the system should not get significantly higher negative publicity and distrust than humans.

References

[1] Lambin P *et al* 2012 Radiomics: extracting more information from medical images using advanced feature analysis *Eur. J. Cancer* **48** 441–46

[2] Kumar V *et al* 2012 Radiomics: the process and the challenges *Magn. Reson. Imaging* **30** 1234–48

[3] Gillies R J, Kinahan P E and Hricak H 2016 Radiomics: images are more than pictures, they are data *Radiology* **278** 563–77

[4] Yip S S F and Aerts H J W L 2016 Applications and limitations of radiomics *Phys. Med. Biol.* **61** R150–66

[5] Parekh V and Jacobs M A 2016 Radiomics: a new application from established techniques *Expert Review of Precision Medicine and Drug Development* **1** 207–26

[6] Hunter L 2013 Radiomics of nsclc: quantitative ct image feature radiomics of nsclc: quantitative ct image feature characterization and tumour shrinkage prediction characterization and tumour shrinkage prediction. *Thesis* University of Texas https://digitalcommons.library.tmc.edu/utgsbs_dissertations

[7] Chicklore S, Goh V, Siddique M, Roy A, Marsden P K and Cook G J R 2013 Quantifying tumour heterogeneity in 18F-FDG PET/CT imaging by texture analysis *Eur. J. Nucl. Med. Mol. Imaging* **40** 133–40

[8] Aerts H J W L *et al* 2014 Decoding tumour phenotype by noninvasive imaging using a quantitative radiomics approach *Nat. Commun.* **5** 1–9

[9] Coroller T P, Grossmann P, Hou Y, Rios Velazquez E, Leijenaar R T H, Hermann G, Lambin P, Haibe-Kains B, Mak R H and Aerts H J W L 2015 CT-based radiomic signature predicts distant metastasis in lung adenocarcinoma *Radiother. Oncol.* **114** 345

[10] Parmar C, Leijenaar R T H, Grossmann P, Velazquez E R, Bussink J, Rietveld D, Rietbergen M M, Haibe-Kains B, Lambin P and Aerts H J W L 2015 Radiomic feature clusters and prognostic signatures specific for lung and head and neck cancer *Sci. Rep.* **5** 11044

[11] Vallières M, Freeman C R, Skamene S R and El Naqa I 2015 A radiomics model from joint FDG-PET and MRI texture features for the prediction of lung metastases in soft-tissue sarcomas of the extremities *Phys. Med. Biol* **60** 5471–96

[12] Peng L *et al* 2018 Distinguishing true progression from radionecrosis after stereotactic radiation therapy for brain metastases with machine learning and radiomics *Int. J. Radiat. Oncol. Biol. Phys.* **102** 1236–43

[13] Hassan I, Kotrotsou A, Bakhtiari A S, Thomas G A, Weinberg J S, Kumar A J, Sawaya R, Luedi M M, Zinn P O and Colen R R 2016 Radiomic texture analysis mapping predicts areas of true functional MRI activity *Sci. Rep.* **6** 25295

[14] Parekh V S and Jacobs M A 2020 Multiparametric radiomics methods for breast cancer tissue characterization using radiological imaging *Breast Cancer Res. Treat.* **180** 407

[15] *Multiparametric imaging* (n.d.). Retrieved March 11, 2022, from https://healthcare-in-europe.com/en/news/multiparametric-imaging.html

[16] Lee G, Lee H Y, Ko E S and Jeong W K 2017 Radiomics and imaging genomics in precision medicine *Precis. Future Med.* **1** 10–31

[17] Bodalal Z, Trebeschi S, Nguyen-Kim T D L, Schats W and Beets-Tan R 2019 Radiogenomics: bridging imaging and genomics *Abdom. Radiol.* **44** 1960–84

[18] Vaidya P *et al* 2020 CT derived radiomic score for predicting the added benefit of adjuvant chemotherapy following surgery in stage I, II resectable non-small cell lung cancer: a retrospective multicohort study for outcome prediction *Lancet Dig. Health* **2** e116–28

[19] Smith C P, Czarniecki M, Mehralivand S, Stoyanova R, Choyke P L, Harmon S and Turkbey B 2019 Radiomics and radiogenomics of prostate cancer *Abdom. Radiol.* **44** 2021–029

[20] Rios Velazquez E *et al* 2017 Somatic mutations drive distinct imaging phenotypes in lung cancer *Cancer Res.* **77** 3922–30

[21] Yip S S F, Kim J, Coroller T P, Parmar C, Velazquez E R, Huynh E, Mak R H and Aerts H J W L 2017 associations between somatic mutations and metabolic imaging phenotypes in non-small cell lung cancer *J. Nucl. Med.* **58** 569–76

[22] Jiang W, Song Y, Sun Z, Qiu J and Shi L 2021 Dosimetric factors and radiomics features within different regions of interest in planning CT images for improving the prediction of radiation pneumonitis Radiomic texture analysis mapping predicts areas of true functional MRI activity**110** 1161–70

[23] Parekh V S and Jacobs M A 2019 Deep learning and radiomics in precision medicine *Expert Rev. Precis. Med. Drug Dev.* **4** 59–72

[24] Parekh V S, Laterra J, Bettegowda C, Bocchieri A E, Pillai J J and Jacobs M A 2019 Multiparametric deep learning and radiomics for tumour grading and treatment response assessment of brain cancer: preliminary results arXiv:1906.04049

[25] Yu H, Wu H, Wang W, Jolly S, Jin J-Y, Hu C and Kong F-M 2019 Machine learning to build and validate a model for radiation pneumonitis prediction in patients with non-small cell lung cancer *Clin. Cancer Res.* **25** 4343–50

[26] Wang W *et al* 2018 IDO immune status after chemoradiation may predict survival in lung cancer patients *Cancer Res.* **78** 809–16

[27] Yu H, Lam K-O, Wu H, Green M, Wang W, Jin J-Y, Hu C, Jolly S, Wang Y and Kong F-M S 2021 Weighted-support vector machine learning classifier of circulating cytokine biomarkers to predict radiation-induced lung fibrosis in non-small-cell lung cancer patients *Front. Oncol.* **10** 601979

[28] Caudell J J, Torres-Roca J F, Gillies R J, Enderling H, Kim S, Rishi A, Moros E G and Harrison L B 2017 The future of personalised radiotherapy for head and neck cancer *Lancet Oncol.* **18** e266–73

[29] Lodwick G S, Keats T E and Dorst J P 1963 The coding of roentgen images for computer analysis as applied to lung cancer *Radiology* **81** 185–200

[30] Haralick R M, Dinstein I and Shanmugam K 1973 Textural features for image classification *IEEE Trans. Syst. Man Cybernet.* **3** 610–21

[31] Li W, Cao P, Zhao D and Wang J 2016 Pulmonary nodule classification with deep convolutional neural networks on computed tomography images *Comput. Math. Methods Med.* **2016** 6215085

[32] Akkus Z, Ali I, Sedlář J, Agrawal J P, Parney I F, Giannini C and Erickson B J 2017 Predicting deletion of chromosomal arms 1p/19q in low-grade gliomas from MR images using machine intelligence *J. Dig.* **30** 469–76

[33] Sato M, Horie K, Hara A, Miyamoto Y, Kurihara K, Tomio K and Yokota H 2018 Application of deep learning to the classification of images from colposcopy *Oncol. Lett.* **15** 3518–23

[34] Esteva A, Kuprel B, Novoa R A, Ko J, Swetter S M, Blau H M and Thrun S 2017 Dermatologist-level classification of skin cancer with deep neural networks *Nature* **542** 115–18

[35] Ypsilantis P P, Siddique M, Sohn H M, Davies A, Cook G, Goh V and Montana G 2015 Predicting response to neoadjuvant chemotherapy with PET imaging using convolutional neural networks *PLoS One* **10** e0137036

[36] Clark K *et al* 2013 The cancer imaging archive (TCIA): maintaining and operating a public information repository *J. Dig. Imaging* **26** 1045–57

[37] Prior F, Smith K, Sharma A, Kirby J, Tarbox L, Clark K, Bennett W, Nolan T and Freymann J 2017 The public cancer radiology imaging collections of the cancer imaging archive *Sci. Data* **4** 170124

[38] Cancer Imaging Archive (n.d.). Retrieved March 12, 2022, from https://cancerimagingarchive.net/

[39] Sollini M, Antunovic L, Chiti A and Kirienko M 2019 Towards clinical application of image mining: a systematic review on artificial intelligence and radiomics *Eur. J. Nucl. Med. Mol. Imaging* **46** 2656–72

[40] Alsalama A 2013 A hybrid recommendation system based on association rules *Masters Theses and Specialist Projects* Western Kentucky University https://digitalcommons.wku.edu/theses/1250

[41] Serban C and Todericiuaa I A 2020 Alexa, what classes do I have today? The use of artificial intelligence via smart speakers in education *Proc. Comput. Sci.* **176** 2849–57

[42] Terzopoulos G and Satratzemi M 2020 Voice assistants and smart speakers in everyday life and in education *Inform Educ.* **19** 473–90

[43] Kumari D and Bhat S 2021 Application of artificial intelligence technology in Tesla—a case study *Int. J. Appl. Eng. Manage. Lett. (IJAEML)* **5** 205–18

[44] Morando A, Gershon P, Mehler B and Reimer B 2020 Driver-initiated tesla autopilot disengagements in naturalistic driving *Proc. 12th Int. ACM Conf. on Automotive User Interfaces and Interactive Vehicular Applications, AutomotiveUI* **2020** 57–65

[45] Juhn Y and Liu H 2020 Artificial intelligence approaches using natural language processing to advance EHR-based clinical research *J. Allerg. Clin. Immunol.* **145** 463–69

[46] Koleck T A, Dreisbach C, Bourne P E and Bakken S 2019 Natural language processing of symptoms documented in free-text narratives of electronic health records: a systematic review *J. Am. Med. Inform. Assoc.* **26** 364–79

[47] Yu K H, Beam A L and Kohane I S 2018 Artificial intelligence in healthcare *Nat. Biomed. Eng.* **2** 719–31

[48] AI platform enables oncologists to practice conversations with terminally ill patients (n.d.) Retrieved March 10, 2022, from https://healio.com/news/hematology-oncology/20220215/ai-platform-enables-oncologists-to-practice-conversations-with-terminally-ill-patients

[49] Building trust in artificial intelligence on JSTOR (n.d.) Retrieved May 6, 2021, from https://jstor.org/stable/26588348?casa_token=wrxedTwP8J8AAAAA%3Ah26Bf2nE3dD-uj-Y3Rz4Wt_pb8R82w0Gw6flRcaWRRu6O8xXR0rPIwBq1rAWqRScnF2nRLwAuKEpZrxLVQ3xCtkIGo-OPe_YeTfx_Ce0W_EvHZIoIKg&seq=2#metadata_info_tab_contents

[50] Bi W L *et al* 2019 Artificial intelligence in cancer imaging: clinical challenges and applications *CA Cancer J. Clin.* **69** 127–57

[51] Gerke S, Minssen T and Cohen G 2020 Ethical and legal challenges of artificial intelligence-driven healthcare *Artificial Intelligence in Healthcare* (Amsterdam: Elsevier) pp 295–336

[52] Judge dismisses data sharing lawsuit against University of Chicago, Google | Fierce Healthcare (n.d.) Retrieved March 12, 2022, from https://fiercehealthcare.com/tech/judge-dismisses-data-sharing-lawsuit-against-university-chicago-google

[53] Dhagarra D, Goswami M and Kumar G 2020 Impact of trust and privacy concerns on technology acceptance in healthcare: an indian perspective *Int. J. Med. Inform.* **141** 104164
[54] Callahan T J, Barnard J G, Helmkamp L J, Maertens J A and Kahn M G 2017 Reporting data quality assessment results: identifying individual and organizational barriers and solutions *EGEMs* **5** 16
[55] Beil M, Proft I, van Heerden D, Sviri S and van Heerden P V 2019 Ethical considerations about artificial intelligence for prognostication in intensive care *Intens. Care Med. Experiment.* **7** 1–13
[56] Shin T (n.d.) Real-life examples of discriminating artificial intelligence | Towards Data Science. Retrieved March 12, 2022, from https://towardsdatascience.com/real-life-examples-of-discriminating-artificial-intelligence-cae395a90070
[57] Obermeyer Z, Powers B, Vogeli C and Mullainathan S 2019 Dissecting racial bias in an algorithm used to manage the health of populations *Science* **366** 447–53
[58] Wang F and Preininger A 2019 AI in health: state of the art, challenges, and future directions *Yearbook Med. Inform.* **28** 16–26
[59] Char D S, Shah N H and Magnus D 2018 Implementing machine learning in health care—addressing ethical challenges *New Engl. J. Med.* **378** 981–83
[60] Researchers say use of artificial intelligence in medicine raises ethical questions | News Center | Stanford Medicine (n.d.) Retrieved May 6, 2021, from https://med.stanford.edu/news/all-news/2018/03/researchers-say-use-of-ai-in-medicine-raises-ethical-questions.html
[61] Shi X Q, Sällström P and Welander U 2002 A color coding method for radiographic images *Image Vision Comput.* **20** 761–67
[62] Bridge to Artificial Intelligence (Bridge2AI) | NIH *Common Fund* (n.d.) Retrieved March 12, 2022, from https://commonfund.nih.gov/bridge2ai
[63] Beane M 2019 Shadow learning: building robotic surgical skill when approved means fail *Admin. Sci. Quart.* **64** 87–123
[64] da Vinci Robotic Surgery Lawsuit: Underreporting and Settlements (n.d.) Retrieved March 10, 2022, from https://drugwatch.com/davinci-surgery/lawsuits/
[65] da Vinci Robotic Surgery Complications—Risks and Malfunction (n.d.) Retrieved March 10, 2022, from https://drugwatch.com/davinci-surgery/complications/

www.ingramcontent.com/pod-product-compliance
Ingram Content Group UK Ltd.
Pitfield, Milton Keynes, MK11 3LW, UK
UKHW051853100926
8556IPUK00005B/611

9 780750 333375